In Clinical Practice

Nick A. Aresti
Manoj Ramachandran
Mark (J.M.H.) Paterson
Matthew Barry
Editors

Paediatric Orthopaedics in Clinical Practice

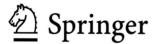 Springer

Editors
Nick A. Aresti, MBBS, MRCS,
PGCertMedEd, FHEA
T&O SpR Percivall Pott Rotation
London
UK

Manoj Ramachandran, BSc,
MBBS, FRCS (T&O)
Paediatric and Young Adult
Orthopaedic Unit
The Royal London and Barts and
The London Children's Hospitals,
Barts Health
London
UK

Mark (J.M.H.) Paterson, FRCS
Paediatric and Young Adult
Orthopaedic Unit
The Royal London and Barts and
The London Children's Hospitals,
Barts Health
London
UK

Matthew Barry, MS, FRCS (Orth)
Paediatric and Young Adult
Orthopaedic Unit
The Royal London and The
London Children's Hospitals,
Barts Health NHS Trust
London
UK

ISSN 2199-6652   ISSN 2199-6660   (electronic)
In Clinical Practice
ISBN 978-1-4471-6767-9   ISBN 978-1-4471-6769-3   (eBook)
DOI 10.1007/978-1-4471-6769-3

Library of Congress Control Number: 2016933134

Springer London Heidelberg New York Dordrecht

Springer-Verlag London Ltd. is part of Springer Science+Business Media
(www.springer.com)

This book is in loving memory of Mark (J.M.H.) Paterson, our dedicated colleague and trusted friend

Dedicated to my wonderful wife-to-be, Stephanie

Nick A. Aresti

For Caroline and my children Max, Fran, Felix and Joe

Matthew Barry

As always, for my wife, Joanna and my daughters Isabel and Mia

Manoj Ramachandran

Mark (J.M.H.) Paterson (1954–2013)

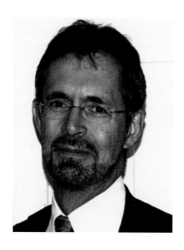

Mark (J.M.H.) Paterson was a key figure in developing Children's Orthopaedic services in East London. He was born in Hong Kong to a family with a history of missionary service. Mark followed his father in studying medicine at the Middlesex Hospital Medical School, graduating in 1977. After house jobs in Norwich, he spent a year working as a Medical Officer in Papua New Guinea where he found himself undertaking varied medical, surgical and even gynaecological work. He then returned to UK training, with junior posts in and around the South-East, and in 1986 was appointed Senior Registrar on the London Hospital training programme. This provided him with opportunity to work at the Royal London and Royal National Orthopaedic Hospitals, and he travelled abroad to gain experience in San Diego and Connecticut. With this experience behind him, he was appointed to the staff of the then London Hospital in 1990 to work initially with Brian Roper in building the services for children. Following Brian Roper's retirement and the ever increasing demand, Mark's role in the department gradually evolved from a consultant with a special interest in children's orthopaedics to a full-time children's practice.

With the increased centralisation of children's services, he soon required additional colleagues and during his career transformed a part-time commitment by one consultant to a department of four children's orthopaedic surgeons. Mark's particular forte was the difficult area of neuromuscular orthopaedics and notably cerebral palsy where his gentle manner, endless patience and understanding, endeared him to his patients, their parents and his colleagues. Despite his hectic work schedule, he was an examiner for the FRCS (Orth) for 5 years and assessor of examiners for a further year. He also examined for the European Board of Orthopaedics and Trauma and for the College of Surgeons in Hong Kong. Additionally he was involved with various surgical societies and President of the Orthopaedic Section of the Royal Society of Medicine 2006–2007. He believed passionately in providing healthcare for the underprivileged and between 2009 and 2012 undertook six charitable missions to Albania where he was involved in the assessment and treatment of children with disability. Mark was an editor of the JBJS journal and also chaired their electronic publishing committee. He helped establish the EFORT/BESBJS Travelling Fellowships, which will continue in his memory. In January 2013, Mark retired from the NHS with the intention of continuing to provide children's services in the independent sector and participating in short-term projects in the third world. Sadly this was not to be due to the untimely intervention of neoplastic disease. He leaves his wife Sarah, whom he met as an undergraduate, and two sons Luke and Jamie. His ever-present, quiet, sensible and unstinting personality will be greatly missed by all of those whose lives he touched.

Introduction

The management of the musculoskeletal conditions of childhood has always been integral to the practice of orthopaedic surgery and indeed the very word reflects this. In 1741 Nicolas Andry stated "..of two Greek Words, viz. *Orthos*, which signifies streight, free from deformity, and *Pais*, a Child. Out of these two words I have compounded that of *Orthopædia.*"

Paediatric orthopaedics as a recognised subspecialty of orthopaedic surgery began to develop in the early 1980s with the formation of various associations such as the European Paediatric Orthopaedic Society (EPOS) in 1982, the British Society for Children's Orthopaedic Surgery (BSCOS) in 1984 and the Paediatric Orthopaedic Society of North America (POSNA) in 1984 and since then, the subspecialty has developed and grown in strength with many surgeons having an exclusively paediatric practice.

Musculoskeletal conditions commonly affect children and in contrast to adult orthopaedics, the surgeon not only has a patient but in addition, the parents and family to manage. It is natural for parents to feel anxious and so the management of their fears and worries is a very important part of the treatment of the child. Physicians working in primary or secondary care who treat children may be presented with a child with an orthopaedic condition. This book will provide concise and authoritative information on all aspects of children's orthopaedics and so give the treating doctor enough information to confidently allay the anxieties of their patients and the parents and to understand when to refer the child to a paediatric orthopaedic surgeon.

Matthew Barry
London, UK

Contents

Contributors

Sulaiman Alazzawi, MBChB, MSc, MRCS T&O SpR Royal London Rotation, London, UK

Nick A. Aresti, MBBS, MRCS, PGCertMedEd, FHEA T&O SpR Percivall Pott Rotation, London, UK

Matthew Barry, MS, FRCS (Orth) Paediatric and Young Adult Orthopaedic Unit, The Royal London and The London Children's Hospitals, Barts Health NHS Trust, London, UK

Alexander Charalambous, MBChB, BSc (Hons), MRCS T&O SpR Royal London Rotation, London, UK

Daud Tai Shan Chou, MBBS, BSc, FRCS (Tr&Orth) T&O SpR Percivall Pott Rotation, London, UK

Sam Heaton, FRCS (Tr&Orth) T&O SpR Royal London Rotation, London, UK

Kyle James, FRCS (Tr&Orth) Paediatric and Young Adult Orthopaedic Unit, The Royal London and Barts and The London Children's Hospitals, Barts Health, London, UK

Lucky Jeyaseelan, MBBS, BSc (Hons), MRCS T&O SpR Percivall Pott Rotation, London, UK

Charlie Jowett, FRCS (Tr&Orth) T&O SpR Royal London Rotation, London, UK

Stephen Key, MA, MBBChir, MRCS (Eng) T&O SpR Royal London Rotation, London, UK

Mark (J.M.H.) Paterson, FRCS Paediatric and Young
Adult Orthopaedic Unit, The Royal London and Barts
and The London Children's Hospitals, Barts Health,
London, UK

Manoj Ramachandran, BSc, MBBS, FRCS (T&O)
Paediatric and Young Adult Orthopaedic Unit, The Royal
London and Barts and The London Children's Hospitals,
Barts Health, London, UK

Zacharia Silk, MBBS, BSc (Hons), MRCS T&O SpR
Percivall Pott Rotation, London, UK

Jagwant Singh, MBBS, MRCS T&O SpR Royal London
Rotation, London, UK

Joanna Thomas, MSc, FRCS (Tr&Orth) T&O SpR Royal
London Rotation, London, UK

Alasdair Thomas, FRCS (Tr&Orth) Post CCT T&O Fellow,
Flinders Medical Centre, Bedford Park, SA

Krishna Vemulapalli, MBBS, FRCS, FRCS (Tr&Orth)
Department of Trauma and Orthopaedics, Barking, Havering
and Redbridge Hospitals, London, UK

Daniel Williams, MBChB, BSc (Hons), MRCS T&O SpR
Percivall Pott Rotation, London, UK

Jonathan Wright, MBBS, BSc (Hons), MRCS T&O SpR
Percivall Pott Rotation, London, UK

Chapter 1
Normal Variants and Self-Limiting Conditions

Mark (J.M.H.) Paterson

Introduction

Many children who are brought to paediatric orthopaedic clinics do not have a pathological condition. Some are simply demonstrating natural variation of appearance, with any measured parameter falling within two standard deviations of the mean. Others may be manifesting either features of a natural developmental process (e.g. bow legs) or minor variations that are likely to correct spontaneously with further growth and development (e.g. persistent femoral anteversion).

Bow Legs

The majority of infants are bow-legged before they stand and walk. It is common for this tendency to persist when the child first starts to bear weight, and the tendency is more marked in early walkers. This bow leg, or genu varum, is characterised by

M.(J.M.H.) Paterson, FRCS
Paediatric and Young Adult Orthopaedic Unit,
The Royal London and Barts and The London Children's
Hospitals, Barts Health, London, UK

N.A. Aresti et al. (eds.), *Paediatric Orthopaedics in Clinical Practice*, In Clinical Practice,
DOI 10.1007/978-1-4471-6769-3_1,
© Springer-Verlag London 2016

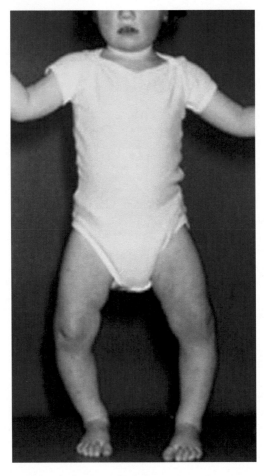

FIGURE 1.1 Bow legs (Reproduced from Benson et al. *Children's Orthopaedics and Fractures*, 2009, Springer)

its bilateral and generally symmetrical nature, and the bowing is usually more apparent in the femoral segment than in the tibial segment (Fig. 1.1). The degree of varus is often seen to increase during the first 6–12 months after standing, before it gradually improves spontaneously between the ages of 2–3 years. This so-called physiological genu varum requires only a clear explanation and reassurance to the parents, and no treatment is needed. Asymmetry, associated torsional problems, and varus which continues to increase beyond the age of 2 years may be pathological rather than a normal variant; the possibility of Blount's disease or rickets should be considered, and radiographs and blood profile for vitamin D deficiency should be obtained.

Otherwise, regular clinical review with estimation of the intercondylar distance at the knees should be undertaken until it is clear that the normal process of spontaneous resolution is occurring.

Spontaneous resolution occurs through differential stimulation of the medial and lateral areas of the distal femoral and proximal tibial growth plates by weight-bearing compressive stresses. Sometimes the compensatory growth stimulation is excessive and parents need to be warned that following the straightening of the bowing, there may be a period of over-compensation into valgus or knock-knee before the legs finally straighten out to around 5–7° of valgus by the age of 4–5 years (Fig. 1.2).

Knock-Knees

Genu valgum or knock-knee (Fig. 1.3) may be a result of overcompensation following a period of genu varum (see above), or it may be a feature of generalised joint laxity (benign hypermobility) particularly in a heavy child. In this latter instance, it may be associated with postural flat feet. Again, if the condition is symmetrical and there is no evidence of vitamin D deficiency, no treatment is required as spontaneous improvement is likely. Regular monitoring of the intermalleolar distance with the child lying on the couch removes the effect of ligamentous laxity, and is an acceptable assessment of progress. Occasionally the knock-knee will persist beyond the first few years of life, and if greater than 12–15° in the older child, may warrant correction by guided growth techniques (hemiephysiodesis).

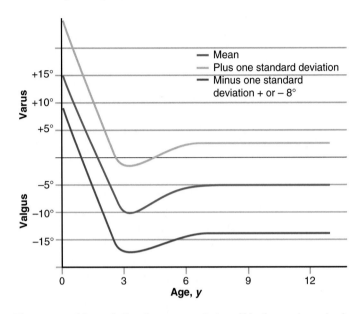

Figure 1.2 Normal development of the tibio-femoral angle in children (Data from Baratz M, Watson AD, Imbriglia JE. *Orthopaedic Surgery the Essentials*. Thieme, 1999)

In-Toeing

The cause of inward turning feet may be at the:

- Hip (persistent femoral anteversion).
- Leg (internal tibial torsion).
- Foot (metatarsus adductus).

The cause may be determined by systematic examination of the entire limb, starting at the hip.

The most common cause is **persistent femoral anteversion**. Neonates have marked proximal femoral anteversion, which gradually decreases through the first decade of life towards the mild anteversion of the adult hip. Persistent femoral anteversion refers to a commonly observed delay in this decrease. This is manifest clinically as a greater range of internal hip rotation

FIGURE 1.3 Radiograph
of idiopathic genu valgum
(Reproduced from Benson
et al. *Children's Orthopaedics
and Fractures*, 2009, Springer)

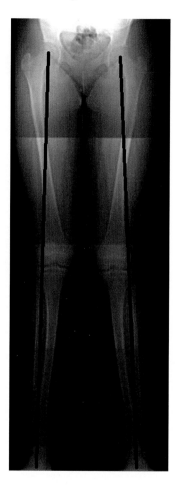

compared with external rotation, giving a resultant comfortable
standing position of some internal rotation and a tendency to
want to sit in a "W-position" (Fig. 1.4). This is best demonstrated
by estimating internal and external rotation of the hips with the
child prone and the knees flexed to act as pointers.

Internal tibial torsion may exist as an isolated phenomenon and tends to decrease spontaneously up to the age of 5–6

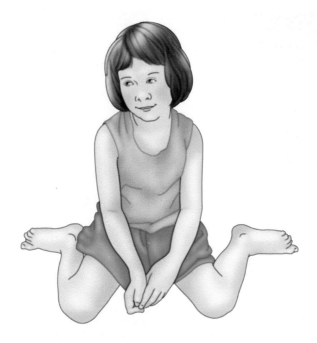

FIGURE 1.4 W position in children

years. It is best demonstrated by estimating the thigh-foot angle whilst the child is still lying prone (Fig. 1.5). No treatment is required in the majority of cases. Persistence of a marked deformity beyond the age of 7 or 8 years may warrant derotation osteotomy at the supramalleolar level.

Metatarsus adductus is a common positional appearance of the foot which may be perpetuated by the infant lying prone with legs tucked up (Fig. 1.6) Again, most of these will remain passively correctable and will resolve spontaneously during the first few years of life. Daily stretches of the medial border of the foot may help to prevent secondary structural contracture, and occasionally serial casting may be needed. However, the majority will not require any treatment. If it becomes fixed or persists beyond 5–6 years of life, simple division of the abductor hallucis is usually sufficient but is rarely necessary. Very rarely, midfoot osteotomies may be indicated.

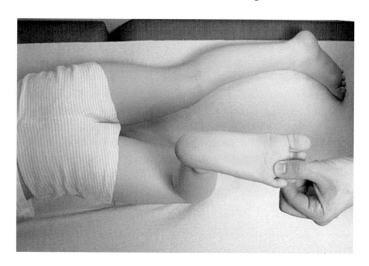

FIGURE 1.5 Estimation of thigh foot angle (Reproduced from Benson et al. *Children's Orthopaedics and Fractures*, 2009, Springer)

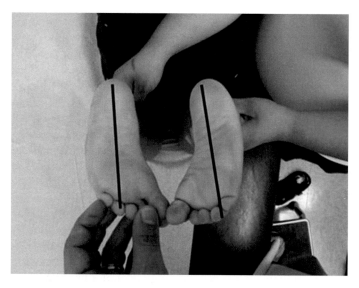

FIGURE 1.6 Example of metatarsus adductus. In this example, the axis of the hind foot differs significantly between the 2 feet (Reproduced from Benson et al. *Children's Orthopaedics and Fractures*, 2009, Springer)

Out-Toeing

This is less common than in-toeing. Close inspection often reveals that this is nothing more than a manifestation of benign flat foot associated with joint hypermobility (see below). Occasionally there may be a predominance of external rotation over internal rotation at the hip joints as a consequence of relative retroversion of the femoral neck. As with femoral anteversion, this is usually within the limits of natural variation and requires no treatment. Children with femoral neck retroversion may be more prone to slipped capital femoral epiphysis (SCFE) if they become heavy in adolescence.

Benign Joint Hypermobility

Some children have a generalised ligamentous laxity, which is not associated with any underlying connective tissue disorder. Such children are able, amongst other features, to hyperextend their elbows and knees, and to bring their thumbs onto the volar aspect of their forearms. This condition is usually familial, with one or other parent recalling similar abilities. They are most likely to present with flat feet, but there may also be a history of an awkward gait or frequent tripping and falling. Walking endurance may be relatively poor, and there may be episodes of non-specific leg pain at night. All these features improve with time and the gradual tightening of the ligaments with growth, and no treatment other than reassurance is required. It is useful to be able to quantify the degree of laxity using the Beighton score (Table 1.1).

Mobile Flat Foot

The presence of mobile postural flat feet (Fig. 1.7) is so common as to be regarded as a variant of normal stance and gait. It is often associated with generalised hypermobility and/or heavy body weight, but neither are prerequisites. The benign postural flatfoot is distinguished from pathological stiff flat

TABLE 1.1 Beighton's modification of the Carter-Wilkinson criteria of hypermobility

Palms flat on the floor with knees extended (1)
Opposition of thumb to flexor aspect of forearm (2)
Hyperextension of fingers parallel to extensor aspect of forearm (2)
Hyperextension of elbows by more than 10° (2)
Hyperextension of knees by more than 10° (2)

Score out of 9 (1 mark for each, including left and right; hypermobile if >6)

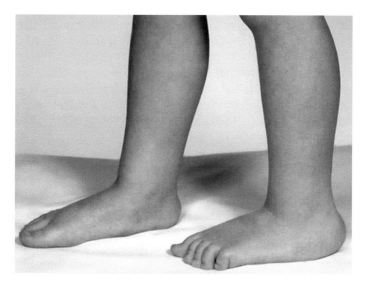

FIGURE 1.7 Example of a flat foot; note the loss of the medial arch (Reproduced from Benson et al. *Children's Orthopaedics and Fractures*, 2009, Springer)

foot by the ability of the child to form a normal longitudinal arch and varus heel when toe-standing or when the hallux is passively dorsiflexed (Jack's test). Normally no treatment is required; there is no evidence for the efficacy of orthotics other than in the occasional instance of medial discomfort on physical activity in the older child. The surgical procedure of arthroeresis (the introduction of a physical block in the subtalar joint to prevent collapse into valgus) does not have wide acceptance in the UK.

Toe-Walking

Some children walk up on their toes from the moment they start to walk. These so-called 'idiopathic toe-walkers' are able to achieve heel-strike if asked to do so, and will stand down on their heels when standing still. They have a normal passive range of dorsiflexion, and examination is normal. It is essential to differentiate these idiopathic toe-walkers from those who are forced to toe-walk because of pathological abnormality. This latter group would include those with spasticity of the calf complexes (e.g. cerebral palsy) and quadriceps weakness (e.g. Duchenne muscular dystrophy). Unilateral toe walking is an indicator of limb length discrepancy and in young children, the possibility of a missed DDH should be considered.

Idiopathic toe-walkers may be managed by maintaining passive ankle range with exercises. Occasionally serial casting may be required to regain lost dorsiflexion range. The use of ankle-foot orthoses in idiopathic toe-walkers is not encouraged. Overlap with conditions such as dyspraxia, dyslexia and autistic spectrum disorder may be seen, and these children do not respond well to constraining orthoses. Ultimately most children will gradually come down on to their heels for walking, under the combined influence of increasing body weight and peer pressure. Rarely, if the tendo Achilles (TA) develops a secondary contracture or if there is a congenitial TA shortening, a percutaneous lengthening (most commonly triple cut) may be indicated.

Chapter 2
The Limping Child

Alasdair Thomas and Manoj Ramachandran

Introduction

The majority of limps will resolve with minimal treatment and no long-term sequelae. Always remember that a limp can also be the primary presentation of far more significant pathology. For the vast majority of cases, a focused clinical history, a well-rehearsed thorough examination and the appropriate utilisation of basic investigations will differentiate between benign and the serious pathologies. The importance of appropriate periods of observation and follow-up cannot be overstated.

This chapter will outline the rationale underlying a safe, systematic approach to the limping child. Key findings in the main differential diagnoses will be given; further detail along with their treatment and outcomes are covered in the relevant chapters.

A. Thomas, FRCS (Tr&Orth)
Post CCT T&O Fellow, Flinders Medical Centre,
Bedford Park, SA, Australia

M. Ramachandran, BSc, MBBS, FRCS (T&O) (✉)
Paediatric and Young Adult Orthopaedic Unit,
The Royal London and Barts and The London Children's
Hospitals, Barts Health, London, UK
e-mail: manojorthopod@gmail.com

N.A. Aresti et al. (eds.), *Paediatric Orthopaedics in Clinical Practice*, In Clinical Practice,
DOI 10.1007/978-1-4471-6769-3_2,
© Springer-Verlag London 2016

Definition

A limp is an abnormality of gait. Common abnormal gaits include:

- Antalgic.
- Trendelenburg.
- Proximal-muscle weakness.
- Spastic gait.
- Short-limbed.

These common gait abnormalities should be recognised and understood, and will be covered briefly in the examination section of this chapter.

General Approach

It is important to have an approach to the limping child so that there is an open mind to the underlying cause. An appreciation of the wide range of causes for a limp based

TABLE 2.1 Causes of a limping child, based on age of the patient

Age	Common conditions
0–5	Transient synovitis
	Septic arthritis
	Osteomyelitis
	Discitis
	DDH
	Toddler's fracture
	Non-accidental injury
5–10	Transient synovitis
	Septic arthritis
	Osteomyelitis
	Discitis
	Perthes' disease
10–15	SCFE
	Septic arthritis
	Osteomyelitis
	Spondylolysis
	Spondylolisthesis

on the anatomical location and the more common causes within certain age groups of children will aid this (Fig. 2.1, Table 2.1).

History

It is important to obtain a complete and precise history, using open questions where possible. The history may well be vague, especially in the case of the younger child. Parents will often find it difficult to describe the exact nature of the limp or provide an accurate timeline of symptoms. It is important not to lead the parents towards a presumptive diagnosis or be overconfident in one's approach as this can lead to greater diagnostic error.

A complete history must include the duration and nature of the limp, the association of the limp with any pain, any episode of trauma which may have been originally dismissed as trivial, recent illness and/or co-current 'red flags' i.e. fever, rigors, malaise, pain poorly responsive to analgesics, night pain (which manifests as night awakening), loss of weight and night sweats. The clinician must be vigilant regarding any recently recorded pyrexia, as swinging pyrexia may be at its trough during the clinical encounter.

Precision regarding the nature of the onset of the limp, whether it is getting better or worse, treatment to date, including use of analgesics (whether simple, strong or NSAIDs), will aid to clarify the severity of the problem and also make the clinician aware that the clinical picture that is being observed may have been affected by that treatment e.g. a controlled pyrexia or a greater range of motion.

Examination

The examination of child can be extremely challenging, especially in a child who is yet to talk. Gaining the confidence of the child and parents is vital.

Standard physiological indices of temperature and pulse should always be recorded, and the standard "look, feel and

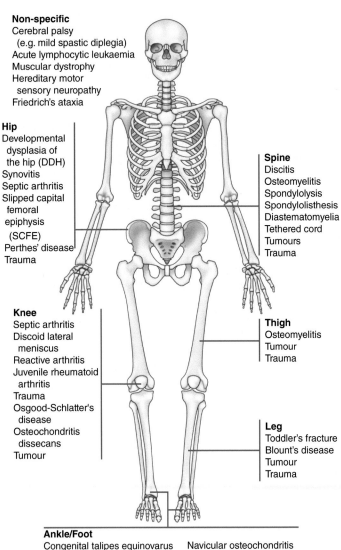

Non-specific
Cerebral palsy
  (e.g. mild spastic diplegia)
Acute lymphocytic leukaemia
Muscular dystrophy
Hereditary motor
  sensory neuropathy
Friedrich's ataxia

Hip
Developmental
  dysplasia of
  the hip (DDH)
Synovitis
Septic arthritis
Slipped capital
  femoral
  epiphysis
  (SCFE)
Perthes' disease
Trauma

Spine
Discitis
Osteomyelitis
Spondylolysis
Spondylolisthesis
Diastematomyelia
Tethered cord
Tumours
Trauma

Knee
Septic arthritis
Discoid lateral
  meniscus
Reactive arthritis
Juvenile rheumatoid
  arthritis
Trauma
Osgood-Schlatter's
  disease
Osteochondritis
  dissecans
Tumour

Thigh
Osteomyelitis
Tumour
Trauma

Leg
Toddler's fracture
Blount's disease
Tumour
Trauma

Ankle/Foot
Congenital talipes equinovarus
  (CTEV)
Osteomyelitis
Juvenile rheumatoid arthritis
Calcaneal apophysitis
  (Sever's disease)

Navicular osteochondritis
  (Kohler's disease)
Tarsal coalition
Pes cavovarus
Accessory navicular
Trauma

FIGURE 2.1 Causes of limping based on site of pathology

move" approach can then be followed. Although the history and observing the child alone may lead to a diagnosis, it is still prudent to examine the child in a complete fashion. The unaffected limb should be examined first so that a comparison can be made and the confidence of the child gained further.

Look

General unobtrusive observation of the child walking and displaying the limp should be the first step. This will require the child to be undressed appropriately.

Gait

Remembering normal gait milestones is important. Children begin to walk independently from 12 to 14 months. This is preceded by crawling or "bum shuffling", the latter of which may delay independent walking. 'Stiff running' may be observed from 16 months. Walking down steps (non-reciprocal) may be observed from 20 to 24 months, and walking up stairs using alternate feet from around 3 years. A mature gait is not usually reached until the age of 7, prior to which a toddler's gait is observed. This consists of a wider base, often a toe to heel foot pattern and a much higher cadence. It may be that a limp cannot be readily appreciated in a slowly ambulating child and may only present itself when he or she walks much quicker or runs.

A systematic approach to the child's gait should be adopted i.e. general cadence, stance and swing phases of each lower limb and then looking up from foot to trunk and back down.

The most common abnormal gait is an antalgic gait with the stance phase being shortened on the painful limb and a reciprocal longer stance phase on the unaffected side. In cases of back or "spinal" pain, a very slow and wary gait may be observed.

A Trendelenburg gait is observed when the abductors have limited function due to weakness, mechanical disadvantage, pain inhibition or a combination of all three. The pelvis is seen to tilt away from the affected side with a compensatory movement of the trunk towards the affected side. When no pain is present, the length of the stance phase is normal; often a Trendelenburg gait will only be seen when the child has walked for a longer period of time.

With proximal muscle weakness, the child will walk with an increased lumbar lordosis and will display Gower's sign (climbing up their body using their hands) on getting up to walk. A spastic gait is most readily recognised when toe walking or scissoring is displayed; however many more subtle signs can be displayed dependent on the muscle groups affected. Again a longer period of observation and asking the child to walk faster may be the only way of revealing the abnormality. A short limb may be recognised from compensatory toe walking on the shortened limb and/or continued flexion of the longer limb at the hip and/or knee.

If the limp cannot be identified, then asking the child to hop with or without assistance may identify the affected limb. With children younger than 3 who usually cannot hop, lifting them up and down from a standing position will often lead to them not placing the affected limb down when landing.

The spine should be inspected for abnormal curvature, swelling, erythema and paraspinal spasm both in the standing and sitting positions. If the child is asked to pick something up from the floor and they have a painful back, they may do so by flexing at the hips and knees keeping their spine stiff and protected.

The vast majority of hip pathology in children will lead to an effusion. This will produce the least pressure and therefore least pain in a position of partial flexion and external rotation; this is the position that children will most often hold their hip when it is the cause of their limp. Both limbs should be inspected carefully for swelling, wasting, erythema and the way in which they are held.

The observation of non-weight bearing is very significant; it can direct the clinician towards a higher risk of a septic arthritis of the hip rather than a transient synovitis and an unstable SCFE compared to a stable SCFE.

Feel

The purpose of palpation is to locate areas of increased swelling, warmth, and tenderness and not to inflict pain. As previously mentioned, if an area has presented itself as the likely source of pathology, other areas should be palpated and moved first. Eye contact is essential for recognising when an area of tenderness has been reached. When swelling is thought to be present, measure the width of the limb at that point and compare it to the other limb.

Move

Often when attempting to examine one joint another is moved; this can be especially confounding in younger children when instructions cannot be followed. Specific methods can be employed to overcome this problem and isolate joints. The greatest amount of information is gained from examining the hip with the patient both supine and prone. Rolling the extended leg gently for rotation at the hip with one hand placed at on the leg and one on the thigh isolates the hip well for testing internal and external rotation. Obligate external rotation of the hip when it is flexed (Drennan's sign) is present even in a mild SCFE that may only have mild radiological signs. Prone examination may help to pick up limitations in internal and external rotation. Sitting the child off the edge of the bed isolates the knee.

Investigations

The most common diagnosis after presenting to an emergency department with a non-traumatic limp is transient synovitis of the hip, with 40% of limps in one series having that diagnosis. In the same series, one patient presented with acute lymphoblastic leukaemia and 30% had no definite diagnosis with no sequelae identified at 1 year. Routine investigations and their corroboration with the history and examination as laid out above will enable the clinician to reliably differentiate between benign and malignant limps, i.e. children that need:

- Outpatient follow up.
- Observation for a short period of time.
- Admission.
- Further urgent investigations and intervention.

With any history of concurrent illness, malaise and/or pyrexia, it is essential to perform an FBC, CRP and ESR. Several series have identified the role and sensitivities of these indices in reaching the correct differential diagnoses.

Standard multi-view radiographs of the areas identified as of concern should be obtained. In an infant and non-verbalising child in which the exact location of the likely pathology cannot be identified, it is justifiable to obtain radiographs of the AP pelvis and the whole lower limb as there is a 20% incidence of occult fracture.

Ultrasound can be very sensitive for identifying effusions in any of the joints and guiding their aspiration. MRI is less practitioner-dependent but requires co-operation of the child and may require general anaesthesia. The role of CT scanning is more limited.

Specific Conditions

Transient Synovitis of the Hip

Transient synovitis of the hip, or irritable hip, is perhaps the most common cause of a limp and hip pain in children. It is a poorly understood pathology that presents with a synovial effusion with a non-inflammatory synovitis. Up to 3% of children are affected.

Risk factors and triggers include:

- Male (2:1).
- Age (4–8 year olds most commonly effected).

- Infection – Approximately 1/3 are in the prodromal period of a viral illness.
- Trauma – Approximately 1/3 follow a minor injury.
- No associate features – Approximately 1/3 follow no specific trigger.

Patients present with a limp and an acute onset of pain, which typically effects the groin or anterior thigh. The limb is normally held in a flexed and externally rotated position, which causes the least amount of pressure on the hip capsule. Adduction and internal rotation cause pain. A low-grade pyrexia may be present. Laboratory results may demonstrate mildly elevated inflammatory markers. A joint aspiration is of no benefit other than to rule out a joint infection.

Transient synovitis is a self limiting disorder which takes around a week to resolve. Treatment is based around bed rest and analgesia, specifically non steroidal anti-inflammatories. The difficulty in managing these patients lies with differentiating a transient synovitis from its differentials, most notoriously an septic arthritis. A CRP of >20 mg/l is the strongest independent predictor of a septic arthritis.

Juvenile Idiopathic Arthritis

Juvenile idiopathic arthritis (JIA) is a term which encompasses a heterogeneous group of typically autoimmune disorders that begin before a patient's 16th birthday and whose symptoms last for at least 6 weeks. Although the symptoms vary with the subtype of JIA, patients will characteristically describe articular pain or tenderness, limitation in movement and joint swelling, unrelated to mechanical disorders. JIA is caused by a combination of environmental factors (e.g. infectious) and immunogenetic susceptibility.

The International League of Associations for Rheumatology published a new classification in 2001 which incorporated historical terms such as 'juvenile chronic arthritis' and 'juvenile rheumatoid arthritis'. This is summarized in Table 2.2.

TABLE 2.2 Juvenile idiopathic arthritis, as classified by International League of Associations for Rheumatology in 2001

Category	Description
Systemic arthritis	This was classically described by George Still in 1897 and is characterised by the triad of: • Arthritis effecting more than 1 joint. • Low grade fever. • Typical erythematous rash. Hepato ± splenomegaly and lymphadenopathy are also possible features. Worrying complications include severe joint destruction and macrophage activation syndrome.
Oligoarthritis	Defined by arthritis involving no more than 4 joints for 6 months. It has a propensity for the lower limbs, the knees and ankles being the most commonly effected. Other features include easy fatigability, atrophied muscles and growth disturbances. Antinuclear antibody is present in around 60% of patients.
Polyarthritis (RF −ve)	An arthritis that affects 5 or more joints in the first 6 months and is immunoglobulin M-rheumatoid factor (IgM-RF) negative. ESR tends to be negative making diagnosis difficult.
Polyarthritis (RF + ve)	As above, an arthritis that affects 5 or more joints in the first 6 months, however IgM-RF is positive. This is the least common of the JIA's. It mimics rheumatoid disease of the adult. It normally presents as a polyarthritis affecting the small joints of the hands and feet. Rheumatoid nodules on the elbows may feature.
Psoriatic arthritis	Defined as arthritis with psoriasis, or arthritis with 2 of the following features: • Dactylitis. • Nail pitting or onycholysis. • Psoriasis in a first-degree relative.

(continued)

TABLE 2.2 (continued)

Category	Description
Enthesitis-related arthritis	This is characterised by arthritis and enthesopathy, i.e. pain or tenderness at the bony insertion of ligaments, tendons, muscles or capsule. The most common site of enthesopathy is the Achilles tendon. This is related to HLA-B 27.
Undifferentiated arthritis	This category caters for those arthritides who do not fall into any of the above categories.

Treatment aims for JIA's include:

– Preserve joint function and mobility.
– Allow normal development of the child.
– Complete control of the disease and prevention of long term problems.

A multi-disciplinary approach is required and involves the use of physical therapy, analgesia, anti-inflammatory drugs, steroids, disease modifying anti-rheumatic drugs (DMARDs) and biological agents.

Conclusion

A limp is the chief presenting complaint for a myriad of conditions. A definitive diagnosis may not be reached during the first clinical encounter and the key to developing a safe approach to this common complaint is to start with an open mind and recognise the serious pathologies that must be excluded. The bedrock is as always a systematic and thorough approach using the key tools of history, examination, simple investigations followed by specialist investigations, and finally appropriate interventions and follow-up.

Key References

Fischer SU, Beattie TF. The limping child: epidemiology, assessment and outcome. J Bone Joint Surg. 1999;81:1029–34.

Halsey MF, Finzel KC, Carrion WV, Haralabatos SS, Gruber MA, Meinhard BP. Toddler's fracture: presumptive diagnosis and treatment. J Pediatr Orthop. 2001;21:152–6.

Leet AI, Skaggs DL. Evaluation of the acutely limping child. Am Fam Physician. 2000;61:1011–8.

Loder RT, Richards BS, Shapiro PS, Reznick LR, Aronson DD. Acute slipped capital femoral epiphysis: the importance of physeal stability. J Bone Joint Surg Am. 1993;75:1134–40.

Petty RE, Southwood TR, Manners P, et al. International League of Associations for Rheumatology classification of juvenile idiopathic arthritis: second revision, Edmonton, 2001. J Rheumatol. 2004;31:390–2.

Chapter 3
Neuromuscular Conditions of Childhood

Mark (J.M.H.) Paterson

Introduction

This chapter covers those conditions in which there are significant musculoskeletal consequences of neurological or muscular pathology. The topics covered are:

- Cerebral palsy.
- Myelodysplasia (spina bifida).
- Poliomyelitis.
- Duchenne muscular dystrophy.
- Hereditary motor and sensory neuropathy.

Cerebral Palsy

Cerebral palsy (CP) is the term given to a group of conditions in which a non-progressive brain lesion at or around birth gives rise to disorders of posture and movement. The lesion may be a discrete focus of haemorrhage or cyst formation, or

M.(J.M.H.) Paterson, FRCS
Paediatric and Young Adult Orthopaedic Unit,
The Royal London and Barts and The London Children's
Hospitals, Barts Health, London, UK

N.A. Aresti et al. (eds.), *Paediatric Orthopaedics
in Clinical Practice*, In Clinical Practice,
DOI 10.1007/978-1-4471-6769-3_3,
© Springer-Verlag London 2016

it may be the result of more diffuse damage from ischaemia or infection. The premature brain is especially vulnerable to ischaemic damage, and babies born under 30 weeks gestation are at high risk of ischaemic hypoxic encephalopathy. There is also a wide range of autosomal recessive inherited syndromes with neurodisability similar to that seen in CP. Overall, CP is relatively common, with an incidence of about 2 per 1000 live births.

As a result of the central lesion, damage to the corticospinal tracts results in impaired control of the spinal reflex arc, which in turn gives rise peripherally to the characteristic movement disorder of spasticity. This is an exaggerated response to the normal stretch reflex. Spastic muscles resist stretch, which is essential for the normal growth and development of muscle. As a consequence, spastic muscle does not grow properly, and contractures and deformity can result (Fig. 3.1). Other movement disorders include athetosis (uncontrolled writhing movements) and dystonia (variable posture). Unlike spasticity, which is a disturbance of pyramidal system function, these latter disorders involve extrapyramidal tracts. The outcome of surgical interventions in these disorders is much less reliable and predictable than that of spasticity.

A child with CP may have:

- Unilateral involvement, as in a stroke (hemiplegia).
- Involvement predominantly of the lower limbs (diplegia).
- Global involvement (quadriplegia).

Although global involvement used to be called quadriplegia, it now tends to be referred to as total body involvement (TBI), in recognition of the important effects on the axial skeleton in the form of scoliosis, and effects on the bulbar system involving swallowing and allied functions.

The role of the orthopaedic surgeon in the management of CP varies according to the extent of neurological involvement. Children with hemiplegia and many with diplegia will be able to walk, and the emphasis here is on treating contractures, foot and upper limb deformities, and torsional deformity in

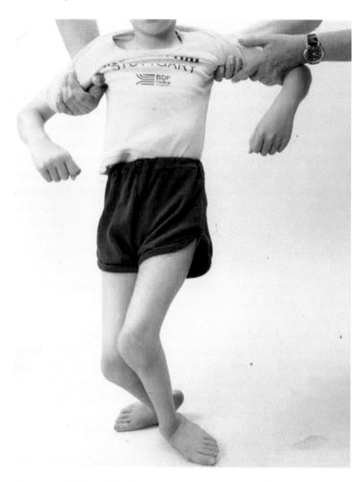

FIGURE 3.1 Bilateral flexion contractures at the knee (Reproduced from Benson et al. *Children's Orthopaedics and Fractures*, 2009, Springer)

the lower limbs. Children with TBI are at particular risk of progressive hip dislocations and scoliosis. However severe the physical disability, it is important to remember that there may be little or no cognitive impairment.

Hemiplegia

This results from a focal lesion in the brain such as a cyst or haemorrhage. The effects are seen on one side of the body in the form of spasticity, which may lead in turn to contractures and deformity. Some muscle groups are involved more than others, giving rise to the typical upper limb posture of adduction and internal rotation at the shoulder, flexion at the elbow, pronation in the forearm, and flexion at the wrist and fingers. In the lower limb, there is typically equinus or equinovarus at the foot and ankle due to involvement of the calf muscles.

Diplegia

This is frequently the result of ischaemic or hypoxic damage to the immature brain and is seen in children who were born prematurely. The most obvious neurological abnormalities are seen in the lower limbs, with the upper limbs and axial skeleton relatively spared. Most of these children have some standing and walking ability, and surgical interventions are directed at maximising their walking potential. Many of them will develop calf and hamstring contractures, and they may have valgus feet and ankles.

Management of both hemiplegia and diplegia in the early years involves joint ranging and stretching exercises to maintain muscle length and encourage muscle growth. Serial casting is a technique that uses the stress-relaxation properties of muscle and tendon to achieve a gradual increase in muscle-tendon length. Children can be helped to adopt a normal gait sequence with the use of ankle-foot orthoses. Tone reduction can be achieved on a temporary basis by use of botulinum toxin, which interrupts motor endplate function by acting as a competitive inhibitor of presynaptic cholinergic receptors. Spasticity may also be reduced by selective destruction of the dorsal spinal roots (selective dorsal rhizotomy) or by continuous intrathecal infusion of baclofen, a tone-reducing drug which is thought to act as a GABA agonist, although its mechanism of action is not fully understood.

Ultimately it may be necessary to lengthen surgically the muscle-tendon unit. Surgery is best avoided in the early years as it interferes with muscle growth. Surgery may also unmask the underlying weakness of the involved muscles, and extensive releases in older heavier children may make it difficult for them to rehabilitate.

It is essential to consider the child as a whole when assessing difficulties with standing and walking. Because of the complex nature of human gait, and the fact that some muscles cross more than one joint and have more than one action, a simple surgical intervention at one level may lead to problems elsewhere. Because of this, instrumented gait analysis has been developed in order to acquire objective gait data, which is used to plan appropriate surgery. This may include lengthening a contracted gastrocnemius or hamstring, stabilising a foot that has been pulled by abnormal muscle tone into a valgus position, or de-rotating a femur that has become internally rotated, again through prolonged unbalanced muscle action. In situations where there is relative overactivity of one muscle, an appropriate tendon transfer may be used to redress the balance. In general, such surgery should be performed in one sitting (single event multilevel surgery) wherever possible, so that the whole limb can be properly balanced and the child has one rehabilitation period.

Total Body Involvement

These children have a wide variety of severe brain abnormalities, including genetic and metabolic defects. They are generally not independent standers or walkers and indeed many will not have the ability to sit or crawl. Many have seizure disorders and as a result of bulbar dysfunction and swallowing problems, many also have feeding difficulties and chest problems, with consequent malnourishment. These factors are of great importance when considering surgical intervention in such children.

The orthopaedic priorities are to prevent and treat progressive hip displacement and scoliosis. Hip reconstruction and spinal correction are major procedures that carry a definite risk to the TBI child. However, a dislocating hip can be a source of severe relentless pain, with associated spasm and deteriorating posture. Consequently the indications for and against surgery have to be weighed up very carefully with all those involved in caring for the child.

Myelodysplasia

These are congenital defects of spinal cord formation, often referred to generally as *spina bifida* (see Chap. 5). The most common form is meningomyelocele, in which there is exposure of the spinal cord and its coverings at a particular spinal level. The incidence of these defects has greatly decreased as a result of the routine administration of folic acid to pregnant women, as well as improved pre-natal screening. Paediatric surgeons are responsible for closure of the neural defect, but orthopaedic surgeons are involved in monitoring development and dealing with the musculoskeletal problems that arise.

Children with these neural tube defects characteristically demonstrate flaccid weakness in muscle groups distal to the lesion. Thus, a child with a myelomeningocele at T12 will have no active muscle in the lower limbs and is likely to be a chair-user. On the other hand, someone with a lesion at L3 is likely to have some hip flexion and knee extension function, and may be expected to walk with an above-knee caliper known as a knee-ankle-foot orthosis (KAFO).

In contrast with cerebral palsy, which is predominantly a motor disorder, children with spina bifida have major problems with sensory loss and dysfunction in their lower limbs. They are at risk of neurotrophic ulceration and careful attention must be paid to the fitting of splints and footwear.

Surgery may be indicated for progressive hip subluxation, joint contractures or rotational deformities.

Poliomyelitis

Despite continued attempts at universal vaccination there is a trickle of new cases of polio every year. Furthermore, orthopaedic surgeons continue to be confronted by the sequelae of infection acquired in the past.

The poliovirus attacks the anterior horn cells in the cord, causing a flaccid lower motor neurone paralysis without any sensory deficit. The typical presentation is of a child with wasting and weakness in one or more limbs who has a history of a severe acute febrile illness in early childhood.

There is some scope for tendon transfer surgery, for example, transfer of a functioning tibialis posterior through the interosseous membrane onto the dorsum of the foot to counteract the dropfoot caused by a paralysed tibialis anterior and toe extensors. In general, however, surgical effort is concentrated on simple bony procedures to correct fixed deformity and enable use of appropriate orthoses.

Quadriceps weakness is common, leading to an inability to maintain knee extension in stance. Affected patients often develop a habit of forcing their knee back into hyperextension to stabilise it, using their hand on their thigh. Such patients may be helped by an extension osteotomy of the knee. Equinus and cavus foot deformities may require either hindfoot fusions or midfoot osteotomies.

Duchenne Muscular Dystrophy

Dystrophies, myopathies and atrophies are generally rare inherited conditions characterised by weakness, muscle imbalance and various deformities, particularly scoliosis (Fig. 3.2). The commonest form of muscular dystrophy is Duchenne muscular dystrophy (DMD). This is an X-linked recessively inherited condition, meaning that it is invariably boys that are affected, with females acting as carriers. The main symptom is progressive weakness that may be apparent from early childhood. The weakness tends to be more marked in the proximal muscle groups, with wasting of the quadriceps

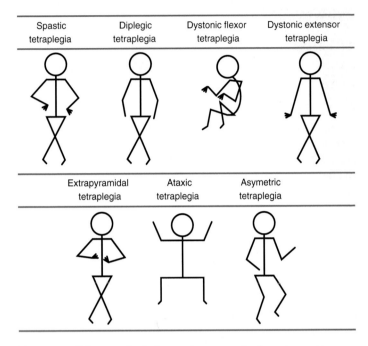

FIGURE 3.2 Diagram depicting various tetraplegia motor patterns

being a key sign (Fig. 3.3). This makes it difficult for affected boys to climb stairs or to get up from a sitting position on the ground without using their hands to "walk" up their thighs (Fig. 3.4). Many children develop toe-walking in order to bring their centre of gravity in front of the knee and thereby compensate for their knee extensor weakness. Progressive loss of walking endurance and fatigue occurs, with eventual loss of walking ability in adolescence. Once a child is a chair-user, there is an increased risk of progressive scoliosis and respiratory problems (Fig. 3.5). With good management of spine, seating and respiratory issues, most boys can now expect to live into their thirties.

The diagnosis is easily confirmed by a creatinine kinase estimation, which will be extremely high. Genetic testing may demonstrate abnormalities of the Xp21 gene.

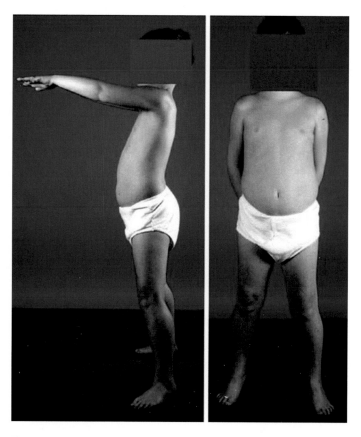

FIGURE 3.3 Example of Duchenne's. Note the equinus at the ankles, pseudohypertrophy of the calf muscles and prominent abdomen (Reproduced from Benson et al. *Children's Orthopaedics and Fractures*, 2009, Springer)

Good orthotic management and carefully-selected muscle releases to address lower limb joint contractures have been shown to delay the time at which these children become obligatory chair-users. Thereafter, any scoliosis must be carefully monitored and surgical correction and stabilisation performed before respiratory function is compromised.

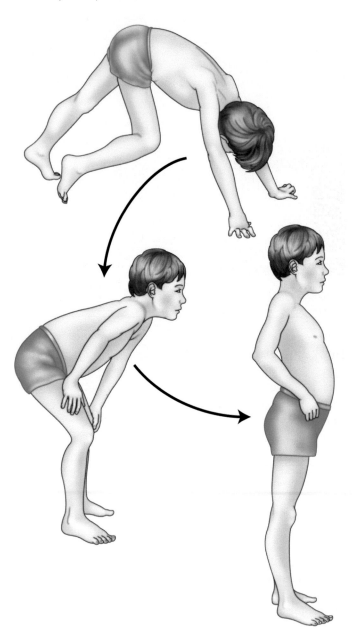

FIGURE 3.4 Gower's sign

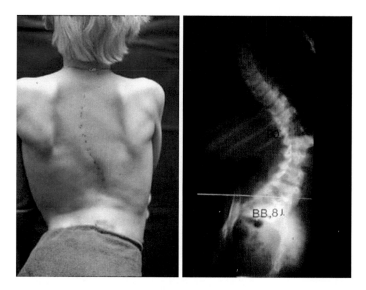

FIGURE 3.5 Severe neuromuscular scoliosis (Reproduced from Benson et al. *Children's Orthopaedics and Fractures*, 2009, Springer)

Becker's Muscular Dystrophy

This is a recessive, X-linked dystrophinopathy, similar to Duchene's. The main distinctions are that the symptoms are less severe and that over 90% of patients remain ambulatory after 40 years. Becker's patients tend to develop delayed gross motor milestones, have pseudohypertrophyied calves and proximal muscle weakness. They are late ambulators, and are perceived as being clumsy and having regular falls. Preservation of neck flexors can help differentiate from Duchenne's. Laboratory studies will reveal raised CK levels and the presence of muscle dystrophin, albeit small levels (compared to Duchenne's where it would be absent). Contractures occur later in life, and life expectancy averages in the early 40's. These patients are at risk of developing cardiomyopathies.

Hereditary Motor-Sensory Neuropathies

There are a large number of these conditions, but by far the most common is HMSN 1 or Charcot-Marie-Tooth disease. In these inherited conditions, there is progressive damage to peripheral nerves in the limbs, resulting in muscle imbalance, weakness and wasting. The characteristic resulting deformity in the lower limbs is a pes cavo-varus, or a foot with an abnormally high arch and in varus. Because of a relatively weak tibialis anterior, the first ray of the foot is pulled plantarward by the unopposed peroneus longus, and this throws the hindfoot into varus. Associated with this are clawing of the toes, secondary contracture of the plantar fascia, and relative overpull of the hindfoot into further varus by a relatively strong tibialis anterior and weak peroneus brevis.

Initially these deformities can be corrected surgically by appropriate soft tissue re-balancing procedures. For these to be successful, the foot must still be supple with mobile joints, and the deformity passively correctable. The Coleman block test (see Chap. 11) is a useful clinical test to differentiate between mobile and fixed deformity.

In the passively correctable foot, transfer of the relatively strong peroneus longus to the weak peroneus brevis, together with plantar fascia release, may be sufficient to re-balance the foot. Additional bony measures such as closing dorsal wedge osteotomy of the first ray or lateral displacement calcaneal osteotomy may be necessary. As the child grows into adult life and the deformities become more severe and rigid, consideration must be given to additional bony procedures such as lateral displacement calcaneal osteotomy and triple fusion (arthrodesis of the joints between talus and calcaneum, talus and navicular, and calcaneum and cuboid). Any residual cavus may require a mid-foot osteotomy.

The pes cavus typical of HMSN 1 may also be seen in conditions of the spinal cord where the cord or cauda equina is stretched, deformed or compressed by tumour or by structural anomalies (tethered cord, diastematomyelia).

Friedreich Ataxia

This is an autosomal recessive ataxia characterised by spino-cerebellar degenerative changes, neuron loss and secondary gliosis in the dorsal root ganglion, spinocerebellar and corti-cospinal tracts, and posterior columns. Patients present with a triad of a progressive spinocerebellar gait ataxia, areflexia and positive plantar response. Other features include weakness, nystagmus, cardiomyopathy and ensuing deformities such as a cavo-varus foot and scoliosis. Around 10% will develop diabetes mellitus.

Chapter 4
Paediatric Upper Limb

Charlie Jowett and Matthew Barry

Introduction

This chapter will review the most frequent congenital and acquired upper limb abnormalities.

These are:

- Shoulder:

    - Obstetric Brachial Plexus Injury (OBPI).
    - Pseudarthrosis of the clavicle.
    - Sprengel deformity.

- Elbow:

    - Congenital radial head dislocation.
    - Radioulnar synostosis.

C. Jowett, FRCS (Tr&Orth)
T&O SpR Royal London Rotation, London, UK

M. Barry, MS, FRCS (Orth) (✉)
Paediatric and Young Adult Orthopaedic Unit,
The Royal London and The London Children's Hospitals,
Barts Health NHS Trust, London, UK
e-mail: matthew.barry@bartshealth.nhs.uk

N.A. Aresti et al. (eds.), *Paediatric Orthopaedics in Clinical Practice*, In Clinical Practice,
DOI 10.1007/978-1-4471-6769-3_4,
© Springer-Verlag London 2016

37

- Wrist:
  - Madelung's deformity.
- Hand:
  - Syndactyly.
  - Camptodactyly.
  - Thumb deformities.

Shoulder

Obstetric Brachial Plexus Injury (OBPI)

This group of conditions occur in around 1 in 1000 live births. Of these, 1 in 10 will be significantly impaired functionally. The injury is usually secondary to traction injuries and is associated with breech deliveries, large babies, prolonged labour, shoulder dystocia and forceps delivery. Patients present with one of the following patterns:

- Erb's palsy: C5,6 lesion ('Waiter's tip deformity').
  The patient presents with the shoulder adducted and internally rotated. The elbow is extended, the forearm pronated and the wrist flexed. This often has a good outcome and 90% recover within 6 months.
- Klumpke's palsy: C8 T1 lesion.
  This is a rare lesion. It presents with weakness in finger flexion and the weakness of the intrinsic hand muscles. The prognosis is worse than that of Erb's palsy.
- Total plexus injury: C5-T1 lesion.
  This has the worst outcome of the OBPI palsies. The patient presents with a flaccid numb arm. Only 40% recover at 6 months.

Around 90% of brachial plexus injuries recover. The function of the biceps brachii is the best indicator of recovery and in babies can be observed if they can bring their hand towards their mouth. A poor prognosis is expected if:

- There has been no recovery after 3 months.
- The injury involves the total plexus.
- Klumpke's palsy.
- The injury is preganglionic.

When examining patients with suspected OBPIs, other differential diagnoses should be considered. These include:

- Clavicle fractures.
- Humeral fractures.
- Arthrogryposis.
- Sprengel shoulder.
- Congenital shoulder dislocation.
- Septic arthritis.

Initial management is non-operative. At 3 months biceps recovery is assessed and an EMG performed if there is no recovery. Surgical management is considered if no biceps function is present at 3–6 months as it is likely that the child will have a residual deficit. Optimal timing of surgery is between 6 months – 1 year. Management options depend on age. A broad guide to what surgical options are indicated at specific ages is summarised below:

- <6 months   Observe.
- 6–12 months   Nerve transfer/graft.
- <2 years   Release contracture of subscapularis/teres. major/pectoralis major.
- 2–5 years   Latissimus dorsi transfer.
- >5 years   Derotational humeral osteotomy.

Pseudarthrosis of the Clavicle

This is a rare condition thought to result either from pressure of the subclavian artery or failure of fusion of the

2 ossification centres of the clavicle. It presents soon after birth with painless swelling of the middle of the clavicle and is almost always on the right side. If it occurs on the left, it is associated with dextrocardia as part of a situs inversus phenomenon. Radiographs demonstrate sclerotic or 'bulbous ends' of the clavicle at the pseudoarthrosis site (Fig. 4.1).

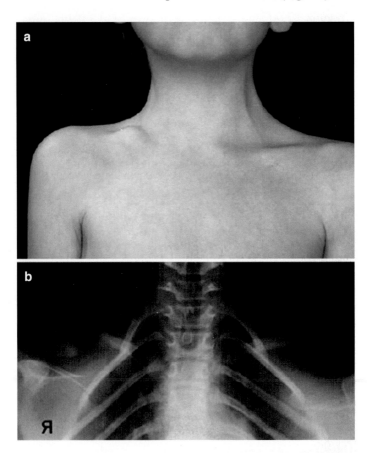

FIGURE 4.1 (a) Clinic photograph of a pseudarthrosis of a clavicle. Notice the prominent lump on the right hand side. (b) Radiograph of the same patient. Notice the prominent sternal half of the clavicle (Reproduced from Benson et al. *Children's Orthopaedics and Fractures*, 2009, Springer)

The main differential diagnosis is a clavicle fracture. This generally presents with pain, a history of a birth disorder and callus on the radiograph.

Surgical options are rarely indicated. Cosmetic issues from the lump are the primary indication for intervention.

Sprengel Deformity

Also known as "congenital elevation of the scapula", this is the most common congenital malformation of the shoulder girdle and has a male to female ratio of 3:1. It is associated with malposition and dysplasia of the scapula. The condition is generally sporadic and most commonly affects the left side, although it may also be bilateral. Associated malformations are often present with this condition. These include scoliosis and upper extremity anomalies. Approximately one third of patients with Klippel-Feil disease will have a Sprengel deformity (Fig. 4.2).

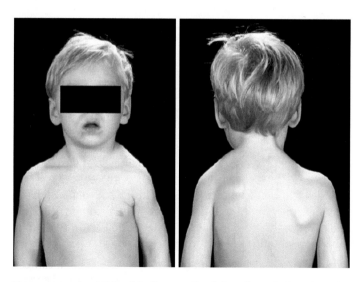

FIGURE 4.2 A child with Sprengel's deformity of the shoulder (Reproduced from Benson et al. *Children's Orthopaedics and Fractures*, 2009, Springer)

Clinically they present with shoulder asymmetry. The affected scapula is elevated and adducted and the inferior pole rotated medially. Scapulothoracic movements may be severely limited. Indications for surgical treatment are when there are significant cosmetic concerns and significant loss of shoulder abduction in children under 6 years of age. During surgery, the dorsal scapular nerve, spinal accessory nerve and the suprascapular nerve are all at risk.

Elbow

To aid with diagnosis and management, knowledge of the secondary ossification centres around the elbow is paramount as the elbow often presents diagnostic problems. The most commonly used mnemonic for the sequence of ossification is CRITOL.

C   Capitellum – 3 years.
R   Radial head – 5 years.
I   Internal (medial) epicondyle – 7 years.
T   Trochlea – 9 years.
O   Olecranon – 11 years.
L   Lateral epicondyle – 13 years.

Congenital Radial Head Dislocation

This is the most common congenital anomaly of the elbow. The aetiology is unknown. The direction of dislocation is anterior in 45%, posterior in 45% and in 10%, there is a lateral dislocation. They are often bilateral and patients have minimal functional limitations. They may become painful in adolescence due to degenerative changes. 60% are related to other abnormalities or syndromes, e.g.:

• Arthrogryposis.
• Larsen syndrome.
• Cornelia de Lange syndrome.
• Nail-patella syndrome.

Clinically the patient has restricted forearm rotation and elbow extension. Radiological findings show that the radial head is dome shaped and there is mild bowing of the proximal ulna. Non-operative treatment is recommended, but if the patient remains symptomatic after skeletal maturity, radial head excision can be considered. Complications associated with earlier resection are postoperative radioulnar synostosis, cubitus valgus deformity, valgus instability and proximal radial migration.

Radioulnar Synostosis (Fig. 4.3)

This condition is usually bilateral and has an autosomal dominant inheritance. It results from failure of segmentation of the radius and ulna. Patients present with a fixed position of the forearm, ranging from neutral rotation to severe pronation. When the condition is mild there is little disability; however when there is severe pronation, it can have a significant impact on activities of daily living.

Attempts at resection of the synostosis to restore rotation have on the whole been unsatisfactory. Rotational osteotomy

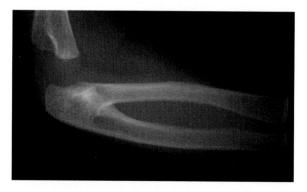

FIGURE 4.3 Radiograph of a proximal radioulnar synostosis, which results from the failure of completion of the distal-to-proximal separation of the forearm mesenchyme

either distal to the synostosis or through the synostosis, fixing the forearm in a functional position have been advocated.

Panner's Disease

This condition begins with necrosis of the capitellum and is followed by regeneration and reossification. The lesion is usually noted in the anterior central capitellum where it is in maximal contact with the head of the radius. Usually the capitellar epiphysis assumes a normal appearance. The mainstay of treatment is non-operative.

Wrist

Madelung's Deformity

This condition is the result of premature fusion of the volar and ulna aspects of the distal radius which results in a progressive ulnar and volar tilt of the distal radial surface with the lunate coming to lie deep between the lower end of the radius and ulna (Fig. 4.4). It is thought to result from volar-ulnar radial physeal arrest. The Vicker's ligament is an abnormal soft tissue tether in the carpal bones between the lunate and distal radius, present in 91% of patients with Madelung's deformity.

Madelung's is an autosomal dominant condition with incomplete penetrance and is more common in females. Differential diagnoses include enchondromatosis (Ollier's), hereditary multiple exostoses, infection and rare generalised dysplasias, such as Leri-Weil dyschondreostosis. The patient is usually asymptomatic and has good function. The wrist is in radial deviation and there is dorsal subluxation of the distal ulna. There is reduced dorsiflexion and supination. It usually becomes apparent during the adolescent growth spurt.

Radiographs of Madelung's deformity demonstrate volar ulna tilt of the distal radius with dorsal subluxation of the

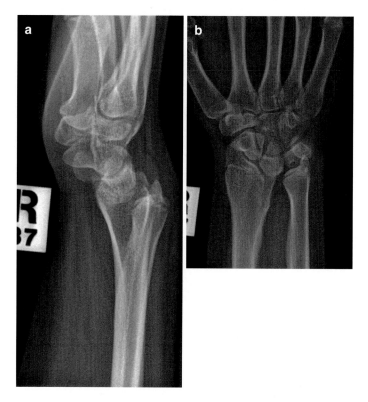

FIGURE 4.4 AP (**b**) and lateral (**a**) radiographs of Madelung's deformity

ulna. The proximal carpal row becomes wedge shaped and the lunate falls into the radio-ulnar gap. Surgery is indicated if there is significant pain and if the deformity starts before the age of 9. Surgical options include:

- Excision of Vicker's ligament and epiphysiolysis of the fused physis with a fat graft.
- Complete epiphysiodeses.
- Epiphysiodesis of the distal ulna.
- Radius (dome) osteotomy ± ulnar shortening.
- Wrist arthrodesis.

Hand

Epidemiology

The incidence of congenital hand deformities has been quoted to be 1 in 626. About 5% of congenital hand anomalies occur as part of a recognised syndrome.

Embryology

Limb development takes place between the 3rd to 8th weeks of gestation. The limb buds occur on the ventrolateral aspects of the embryo and are covered with a thick layer of ectoderm, termed the apical ectodermal ridge (AER). A number of fibroblast growth factors (FGFs) are expressed by the AER, contributing to limb development.

The homeobox genes (HOX) encode transcription factors critical for limb development. Subsequently ossification of the phalanges takes place antenatally while the carpal bones ossify postnatally. Ossification of the congenitally deformed limb is delayed.

Aetiology

The causes of congenital anomalies can be subdivided into genetic, environmental and unknown.

Classification of Congenital Hand Anomalies

Swanson's classification system is the most widely used. It is based on clinical and morphologic appearance:

- Type I: Failure of formation.

  - Transverse arrest – This can be at any level from shoulder to phalanx.

- Longitudinal arrest – May be:
  - Preaxial (varying degrees of hypoplasia of the thumb or radius).
  - Postaxial (varying degrees of the hypothenar eminence or ulnar hypoplasia).
  - Central (leading to cleft hand).

- Type II: Failure of differentiation.
  - May be soft tissue (inc. syndactyly), skeletal (including synostoses) or tumorous (including neurogenic or vascular malformations).

- Type III: Duplication.
  - May apply to digits (polydactyly), whole limbs or mirror hands.

- Type IV: Overgrowth.
  - Includes hemihypertrophy (asymmetric limb size) and macrodactyly (digit enlargement).

- Type V: Undergrowth.
  - Includes radial (thumb) hypoplasia, brachydactyly (shortening of digits) and brachysyndactyly (shortening of digits with webbing).

- Type VI: Congenital constriction band syndrome.
  - Intrauterine bands lead to constriction of foetal tissue, in severe cases resulting in amputation distal to lesion.

- Type VII: Generalised skeletal anomalies.

Types of Hand Anomalies

The most common congenital hand anomalies are syndactyly and polydactyly. These occur in approximately 1 in 3000 live births.

- Syndactyly – i.e. two or more digits are fused together (Fig. 4.5).

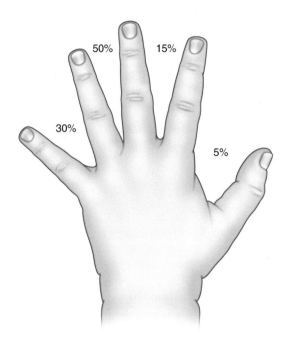

FIGURE 4.5 The frequency of syndactyly of the digital clefts

- Complete vs incomplete; complete syndactyly extends to the tips of the fingers whereas incomplete syndactyly does not.
- Simple vs complex: Simple syndactly refers to situations in which only skin joins the affected digits. Complex syndactyly describes shared or conjoined bone, joints or tendons.

• Polydactyl – i.e. an extra digit.

- Preaxial (radial) polydactyl - Refers to thumb, or first digit duplications (most common).
- Post axial (ulna) – Refers to little finger duplications.
- Central – Refers to duplications of the 2nd, 3rd and 4th digits.

- Camptodactyly – i.e. flexion (most common) or extension deformities, which usually occur in the PIPJ of the little finger.
- Clinodactyly – i.e. a curvature of a digit in the radioulnar plane.

    - Common in patients with Down's syndrome/trisomy 21 (up to 25%).

- Thumb duplications – The Wassel classification is used to describe preaxial polydactyly based upon the level of the thumb duplication from distal to proximal.
- The most common congenital amputation in the upper limb is the elbow amputation with an estimated incidence of 1 in 20,000 live births.

Acquired Hand Deformities

- Trigger thumb – This pathology normally develops between 3 and 6 months of age. It is most commonly locked in flexion at the interphalangeal joint and results from thickening of the flexor pollicis longus (FPL) tendon where it enters the flexor tendon sheath, just proximal to the A1 pulley. The thickening can be felt as a nodule (Notta's nodule) at the level of the metacarpophalangeal joint. It is bilateral in 25%. About 50% of cases will resolve within the first 2 years of life. Spontaneous resolution after the age of 2–3 is unlikely and therefore surgery is indicated. Release of the A1 pulley will correct the problem.
- Clasped thumb – The thumb is held flexed and adducted into the palm at the metacarpophalangeal joint and lacks active extension. The abnormal anatomy includes attenuation or deficiency of the extensor pollicis longus and/or brevis. It is associated with 1st web space, adductor pollicis and interosseous contractures. There are two types: supple and complex. Initially the treatment is splinting for both. In complex cases, surgery may be required.
- Trigger fingers – These can be caused by anatomic abnormalities of the flexor tendons or functional imbalance

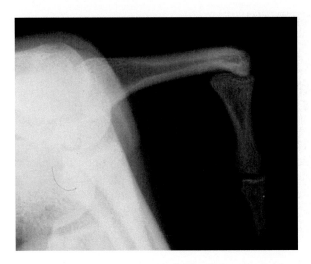

FIGURE 4.6 Camptodactyly with secondary deformity of the head of the proximal phalanx (Reproduced from Benson et al. *Children's Orthopaedics and Fractures*, 2009, Springer)

between the profundus and superficialis tendons. Adequate treatment requires exploration of the flexor mechanism as well as release of the A1 pulley.

- Camptodactyly (Fig. 4.6) – Angulation in the flexion/extension plane. This anomaly can be congenital (as previously mentioned) or acquired. The acquired form presents in adolescence and is more common in females. In both forms, the ulnar fingers are more affected. It is caused by abnormalities in the insertion of extrinsic or intrinsic flexor tendons and a presumed imbalance between flexor and extensor forces in the digit. Night splints for prolonged periods are the standard treatment. Daytime passive stretching is important. Surgery is only considered in severe cases.

- Kirner's deformity (Fig. 4.7) – This is a radial and palmar angulation of the distal phalanx caused by a disruption of the radial and palmar part of the distal and phalangeal growth plate. Surgery is only usually considered for cosmetic reasons.

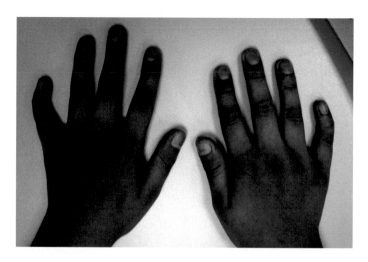

FIGURE 4.7 Kirner's deformity with palmar angulation of the distal phalanx (Reproduced from Benson et al. *Children's Orthopaedics and Fractures*, 2009, Springer)

- Macrodactyly – This is focal gigantism with a disproportionately big digit or digits. It is thought to be a hamartomatous enlargement of soft tissue and underlying bone. It may be present at birth or during infancy. Non-operative treatment is not effective. Surgical treatment involves debulking the affected digits and trying to preserve function. Amputation may be considered in the case of grossly enlarged non-functional digits, as this may improve both cosmesis and function.

Key Reference

Swanson AB. A classification for congenital limb malformations. J Hand Surg Am. 1976;1(1):8–22.

Chapter 5
Paediatric Spine

Nick A. Aresti and Matthew Barry

Introduction

Spinal problems in children are uncommon and this chapter aims to outline the conditions that can affect the paediatric spine and to highlight the rare but serious differentials.

Definition

Some of the more common disorders to be discussed are defined below:

- Spondylolisthesis – The forward translation of a vertebra relative to its caudal segment (Fig. 5.1).

N.A. Aresti, MBBS, MRCS, PGCertMedEd, FHEA
T&O SpR Percivall Pott Rotation, London, UK

M. Barry, MS, FRCS (Orth) (✉)
Paediatric and Young Adult Orthopaedic Unit,
The Royal London and The London Children's Hospitals,
Barts Health NHS Trust, London, UK
e-mail: matthew.barry@bartshealth.nhs.uk

N.A. Aresti et al. (eds.), *Paediatric Orthopaedics in Clinical Practice*, In Clinical Practice, DOI 10.1007/978-1-4471-6769-3_5,
© Springer-Verlag London 2016

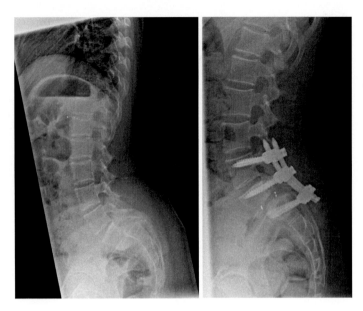

FIGURE 5.1 Lateral radiographs of a high grade spondylolisthesis, both pre and post-op

- Spondylolysis – A defect in the pars interarticularis (the area of bone between the superior and inferior articular processes).
- Scoliosis – Lateral curvature of the spine with an associated rotational element.

Epidemiology/Aetiology

Under the age of 12, back pain is rare and commonly associated with either a tumour or infection. There must be a high index of suspicion – look for red flags clinically, biochemically and radiographically. After the age of 12, pain is more commonly non-specific and less likely to be due to significant pathology.

Assessment

Assessing a younger child with back pain is difficult as symptoms and signs are subtle, but may include:

- A limp.
- Reluctance to weight bear.
- Localised spinal pain/tenderness.
- Constitutional symptoms such as fever, pyrexia and raised inflammatory markers.

Examination

- Younger children may have to be examined supine to assess for alignment, spinal stiffness, muscle wasting or spasm.
- Older children can be examined standing, with deformities exaggerated when flexed forward.

Spondylolysis and Spondylolisthesis

Spondylolisthesis is the movement of one vertebra relative to another, and is, more precisely, the forward translation of a vertebra relative to its caudal segment. The main causes in the paediatric population include:

- Congenital or dysplastic.

  - Dysplastic or congenital abnormality at the L5/S1 facet, with forward translation of the L5 vertebra on S1.
  - More common in girls.
  - Can present following growth spurts in adolescence.

- Isthmic.

  - This is due to a spondylolytic lesion, i.e. an anatomic defect of the pars interarticularis.
  - The lesion is present in around 5% of children, half of which go on to develop spondylolisthesis.

  – Repeated trauma leads to repeated micro-fractures, which may not heal or may heal with an elongated pars.

Risk factors for spondylolysthesis include vigorous exercise, participation in competitive sports involving repetitive lumbar extension, and Scheuermann's disease. The incidence may be as high as 47% in young divers and gymnasts. There is a strong genetic element with boys being affected twice as much as girls.

Symptoms and Signs

Patients tend to experience low back, buttock or thigh pain, which is exacerbated by activity. In patients with isthmic type spondylolysthesis, radicular symptoms are rare but may be due to either hypertrophic callus formation at a pars defect or due to stretching of the nerve in high grade slips. Sciatica is reported by around 50% of patients. In patients with the congenital type, neurological symptoms are more common due to anterior translation of the L5 vertebral body with intact posterior elements, leading to compression of the L5 and sacral nerve roots.

Examination

The examination findings may be the result of localised pain, compensatory muscle or skeletal imbalance, and due to neurological abnormalities. The patient may experience pain on deep palpation of the lesion. There may be an increase in lumbar lordosis – the hamstring, iliopsoas and paraspinal muscles may contract, rotating the pelvis to arch the thoracolumbar spine into maximum lordosis with an exaggerated kyphosis at the sacrum.

Investigations

- Plain radiographs – taken with patients standing to exaggerate any deformity.
- 45° oblique X-rays may be useful in identifying pars defects.
- AP and lateral views of the whole spine may identify a secondary scoliosis caused by muscle imbalance.
- CT scan – the bony architecture can be visualised more readily on CT however the defect can be missed as it may be in the plane of the images. The images should be reformatted into a different plane ("reverse gantry angle").
- MRI – is invaluable in visualizing the neural structures in cases of spinal stenosis and for assessing the corresponding discs. An MRI is indicated in the presence of abnormal neurology.

Classification

The Meyerding classification is most commonly used.

- Grade I – 0–25% slip.
- Grade II – 26–50% slip.
- Grade III – 51–75% slip.
- Grade IV – 76–99% slip.
- Grade V – 100% slip (spondyloptosis).

Treatment

Non-operative Treatment

Asymptomatic slip – monitor over 3–6 months with serial radiographs to ensure the slip is not progressing.

Symptomatic Slip

- Most patients with low grade slips will respond to non operative treatment.

  - Activity modification with physiotherapy.
  - Immobilisation in a brace for 6–12 weeks may aid symptom control.
  - Monitor with serial radiographs to ensure the slip is not progressing.

Surgical Options

- Low grade spondylolisthesis (<50% slip) or spondylosis.

  - Surgery is indicated in patients in whom there is.

    - Failure of non-operative management.
    - Progressive slip on serial X-rays.
    - Neurological deficit for >6 months.

An L5/S1 slip is generally fused, although more proximal lesions can be treated with repair of the pars defects so long as the lesion is reducible and the vertebral disc is intact.

- High grade spondylolisthesis (>50%).

  - Operative stabilisation: fusion with or without instrumentation.

Complications

Complications following surgery include:

- Neurological injury.

  - Cauda equina syndrome must always be excluded through a thorough neurological evaluation.

- Failure of the metalwork/hardware.
- Progression of the slip.
- Pseudoarthrosis.

Synopsis

Spondylolisthesis is a fairly common cause of back pain in children and adolescence. High grade slips or those who are persistently symptomatic may be managed operatively.

Scoliosis

Spinal deformity may be due to an intrinsic problem or secondary to an extrinsic factor such as a leg length discrepancy or infection. Resolution of the extrinsic cause will generally correct the spinal deformity although long standing secondary causes can result in fixed spinal deformity.

The intrinsic causes of spinal deformity are classified by the cause (Scoliosis Research Society):

1. Idiopathic.
2. Congenital.
3. Neuromuscular.
4. Neurofibromatosis.
5. Mesenchymal disorders.
6. Trauma.
7. Infection.
8. Tumours.
9. Miscellaneous.

The most common cause of scoliosis in the paediatric population is idiopathic.

Definition

A scoliosis is defined as a fixed lateral curvature of the spine associated with rotation of the vertebrae.

Idiopathic scoliosis can develop at any time during the maturation of a child's spine. Previously, scoliosis was classified as infantile, juvenile or adolescent. These periods were thought to correspond to periods of accelerated spine growth but perhaps more important, the risk of developing serious cardiopulmonary compromise is far greater in children who develop scoliosis below the age of 5. As such, idiopathic scoliosis is now more conveniently classified as:

- Early onset – scoliosis develops before the age of 5.
- Late onset – scoliosis develops after the age of 5.

Late Onset Idiopathic Scoliosis

Late onset scoliosis rarely causes morbidity but does impact on the child's life and cosmesis. Although there is a fairly even gender split with small curves, female patients predominate in the 'severe curve' category.

Symptoms/Signs

Patients principally present with cosmetic issues. Significant back pain is uncommon.

Examination

Patients should be examined standing and from behind.

- Abnormal coronal balance.
- Shoulder height asymmetry.
- Waist contour asymmetry.
- Hip prominence.
- Forward flexion – the curve will become more apparent with prominence of the spine at the level of the maximum curve (Adam's forward bending test).
- Lower limb neurology must be fully evaluated.
- Assessment of abdominal reflexes. The reflex is characteristically absent on the same side as the curve convexity.

Investigations

Plain radiographs form the mainstay of investigations. Standing AP and lateral radiographs of the whole spine allow evaluation of the degree of the deformity (Cobb angle.) (Fig. 5.2).

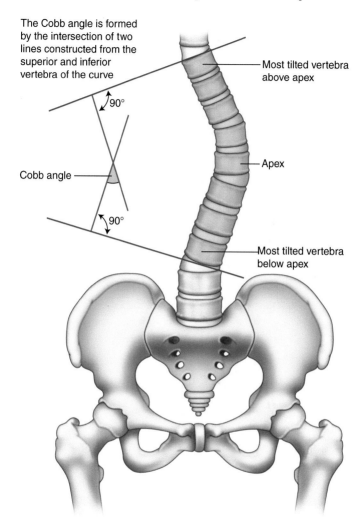

The Cobb angle is formed by the intersection of two lines constructed from the superior and inferior vertebra of the curve

Most tilted vertebra above apex

90°

Apex

Cobb angle

90°

Most tilted vertebra below apex

FIGURE 5.2 Calculation of the Cobb angle

Assessment of skeletal maturity is important to determine the potential for curve progression. At skeletal maturity, the curve will not progress to any further significant amount.

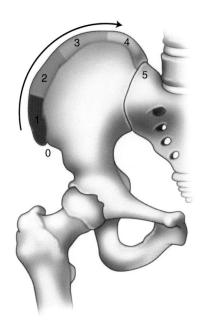

The Risser grading system divides the iliac crest apophysis into four quarters. The fusion of the crest in a lateral to medial manner can be identified radiographically and used to quantify the skeletal maturity.

The Risser stage corresponds to the degree of ossification, i.e. Stage 0 = none, to stage 5 = complete fusion.

FIGURE 5.3 The Risser grading system

Skeletal maturity in girls is approximately 18 months to 2 years after menarche and radiologically, spinal growth ceases at Risser grade 4 (Fig. 5.3).

Differential Diagnosis

Perhaps the important fact to consider in patients in whom you have identified a scoliosis, is its aetiology. It is important to distinguish between those which are non-idiopathic or congenital scolioses. These have very different treatment algorithms and should be considered separately.

Scoliosis "red flags"
- Atypical curve pattern.
- Rapid curve progression.
- Painful scoliosis.
- Abnormal neurology.

The presence of any these factors should raise the suspicion of a tumour, syrinx or infection. MRI imaging is mandatory

Management

Non-operative Treatment

Any patient with an idiopathic scoliosis should be monitored with radiographs approximately every 6 months.

- Observation

   - Curves <30° or skeletally mature patients.

- Bracing

   - Bracing may slow or even stop the progression of the curve, but will not improve the curve. The brace should be worn for 23 h per day, until spinal growth ceases. Patient compliance with this may be a problem. The indications for bracing are:

      - Curves that progress >25° whilst under observation.
      - Curves >30° in skeletally immature patients.

Operative Treatment

Surgery is generally indicated for curves of greater than 40°. Posterior spinal fusion with instrumentation is the most common surgical intervention. A combined (front & back) fusion is reserved for more severe deformities (>75°).

Surgical correction of the deformity aims to produce a well-balanced spine in the coronal and sagittal planes. Fusion below L4 level is associated with low back pain and should be avoided if possible.

Follow-Up

Patients should be followed up to skeletal maturity and the curve monitored clinically and radiologically every 6–12 months.

Complications

Non-operative Management

- Back pain.
- Unfavourable cosmetic appearance.

Operative Management

- Iatrogenic neurological injury.
- Non union.
- Implant failure.
- Loss of lumbar lordosis leading to low back pain (flat back syndrome).
- Continued anterior growth in posteriorly fused spines leading to rotation and deformity (crankshaft phenomenon).

Early Onset Idiopathic Scoliosis

Early onset idiopathic scoliosis can result in compromised cardiopulmonary function secondary to inhibition of growth of the primary pulmonary arterioles and alveoli as a result of the spinal deformity.

Most curves resolve with time, with only around a quarter progressing and requiring treatment.

Predictors of curve progression include:

- Younger age of onset of curve.
- Right thoracic curve pattern.
- Low birth weight.

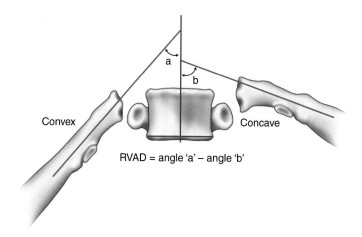

Convex

Concave

RVAD = angle 'a' – angle 'b'

FIGURE 5.4 Estimation of the rib-vertebra angle difference (RVAD)

- Delayed motor mile stones.
- Female sex.
- Rigid curve.
- Rib-vertebra angle difference (RVAD) greater than 20° (Fig. 5.4).

Symptoms/Signs

The clinical evaluation is much the same as in late onset scoliosis but relevant points in this younger age group include:

- Birth history: breech presentation, low birth weight, low tone and prematurity are all associated with a higher incidence of early idiopathic scoliosis.
- Delayed motor milestones.
- Associated conditions:

  - Plagiocephaly.
  - Developmental dysplasia of the hip.
  - Inguinal hernia.
  - Congenital heart disease.

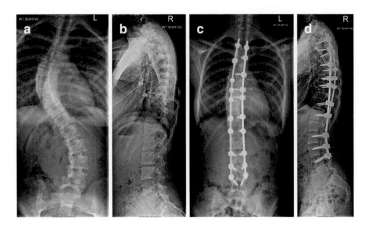

FIGURE 5.5 Pre (**a**, **b**) and post (**c**, **d**) correction radiographs of an idiopathic scoliosis

Imaging is much the same as late onset scoliosis (Fig. 5.5). An underlying neurological abnormality is high in patients who present with curves >20°, so whole spine MRI should be considered. Cardiopulmonary function should be assessed and monitored.

Management

Non-operative

- Cobb angle of <20° and RVAD <20°.
  - Physiotherapy, casting and bracing.

Operative

- Cobb angles >20–35° and RVAD >20° with overlapping ribs and vertebrae ("phase 2") have a high risk of progression and surgical treatment should be considered.
- Cobb angles of >35°.

The main surgical options include definitive fusion and the use of growing rods.

Synopsis

Early onset scoliosis can result in compromised cardiopulmonary function and late onset scoliosis can result in a significant cosmetic deformity. Management includes initial observation and if the curve progresses to a significant angle, surgical intervention may be required.

Spinal Dysraphism

This is a global term that is used to describe failure of closure of the neural tube and encompasses many different pathologies, some of which are considered below.

Spina Bifida

Spina bifida is a term that describes a group of neural tube defects that are caused by failure of formation of the vertebral arches. Deformity leads to nerve abnormality and denervation of organs supplied accordingly. Two subtypes exist:

- Spina bifida cystica – where a cyst forms and is visible.

  - Myeloschisis – the severest form, which involves herniation of the spinal elements in a flattened, plate-like mass of nervous tissue with no overlying skin or membrane.
  - Myelomeningocele – fluid filled sac that contains the dysplastic spinal cord and nerve roots (depending on the level), which is lined by dura and acarchnoid.
  - Meningocele – a protrusion of dura and arachnoid. The cord itself remains confined within the vertebral arches.

- Spina bifida occulta – where the defect is covered and hence hidden from clinical examination. The neural elements remain within the spinal canal however the spine is bifid due to failure of formation of the vertebral arches, and failure of separation of the skin from the neural tissue may lead to a dimple, cleft of hair, pigmentation or a lipoma.

Spina bifida causes a range of problems and treatment is best conducted via a multidisciplinary team. Orthopaedic issues include:

- Spinal deformity.
- Pathological fractures.
- Deformity (generally of the muscles innervated by nerve roots distal to the lowest functioning nerve root).
- Hip dysplasia.

Tethered Cord

A tethered cord is a syndrome of various aetiologies whereby abnormal tension in the spinal cord leads to abnormal neurological function. A tethered cord may be primary whereby it occurs in isolation, or secondary whereby it occurs as a result of another pathology, such as a myelomeningocele, filum terminale lipoma or trauma and ensuing scar formation.

Diastematomyelia

Diastematomyelia describes a condition whereby a sagittal cleft (formed by an osseous, cartilaginous, or fibrous septum) splits the spinal cord, conus medullaris or filum terminale. When the cord is involved, each of the two resultant hemicords contain part of the central canal, a dorsal root and a ventral root, with resultant neurological abnormlaity.

Syringomyelia

Syringomyelia is the formation of a fluid filled cavity (syrinx) within the spinal cord that partially obstructs CSF flow. Aetiologies include abnormalities at the cranio-cervical junction, trauma, tumour and infection. Scoliosis, Klippel-Feil deformity and Charcot joints are all associated orthopaedic conditions.

Chapter 6
Developmental Dysplasia of the Hip

Jonathan Wright and Kyle James

Introduction

Developmental dysplasia of the hip (DDH) represents a spectrum of disorders, which can affect the acetabulum and proximal femur. These can range from a subtle uncovering of the femoral head within the acetabulum, to a complete dislocation of the hip, with degrees of instability between the two extremes.

Normal development of the hip requires interaction between the femoral head and the acetabulum. A concentrically reduced, spherical femoral head will allow normal growth of the acetabulum, whereas an unstable hip may lead to progressive dysplasia and complete dislocation of the hip.

J. Wright, MBBS, BSc (Hons), MRCS
T&O SpR Percivall Pott Rotation, London, UK

K. James, FRCS (Tr&Orth) (✉)
Paediatric and Young Adult Orthopaedic Unit, The Royal London and Barts and The London Children's Hospitals, Barts Health, London, UK
e-mail: kyledimitrijames@gmail.com

N.A. Aresti et al. (eds.), *Paediatric Orthopaedics in Clinical Practice*, In Clinical Practice, DOI 10.1007/978-1-4471-6769-3_6, © Springer-Verlag London 2016

Epidemiology

Up to 1 in 60 babies demonstrate clinical instability of the hips at birth. Around 60% of these will be stable at 1 week and around 88% stable by 2 months. Ultrasound may demonstrate subtle dysplasia, not detectable clinically, that may not have been included in the historic literature.

The reported incidence of DDH varies widely according to geographic and racial background. Rates of hip dislocation in northern Europe are approximately 1–5 in 1000 live births. Reports in the Native American group are 30 times higher, whereas in the African Bantu group, no cases of hip dislocation were seen in a group of 16,678 children.

DDH is seen more frequently in girls than boys (80% girls) with this proportion largely maintained across ethnic groups. It affects the left hip more frequently than the right (64%).

Aetiology/Pathology

The aetiology of DDH is multifactorial; the development of the hip can be affected by both intrauterine and post-natal factors. Twin studies have demonstrated that there is a genetic component with greater rates of DDH seen in the identical twin of an affected child (34%) than in non-identical twins (8%). With an affected child, the risk of DDH in subsequent children being affected has been reported as 6%, an affected parent leads to a risk of 12% and with both an affected child and parent, the risk is 36%. Increased ligamentous laxity and a tendency for a shallow acetabulum have both been suggested as inheritable factors increasing susceptibility to DDH.

The intrauterine environment and positioning can both play a role in the risk of DDH. Oligohydramnios, high birth weight and first-born child demonstrate increased risk, through crowding and restriction of the foetus and due to the nulliparous uterus. Breech positioning in the last 4 weeks of gestation is associated with up to 17 times the risk of DDH. Other "packaging disorders" show association with risk of DDH, such as metatarsus adductus, talipes calcaneovalgus, congenital hyperextension of the knee, infantile skeletal skew (curvature of the spine) and torticollis. There is no association with idiopathic clubfoot. Teratological causes of DDH include arthrogryposis and neuromuscular disorders, such as myelomeningocoele. These are often associated with early intrauterine dislocation of the hip and are frequently irreducible.

As may be expected with an evolving condition, the positioning of the child postnatally plays a role in the development of the hip. Swaddling (as traditionally used by some Native Americans) increases the risk of dysplasia through holding the hip in adduction and extension. Conversely, in areas where children have been traditionally carried with their legs abducted around the mother's back (such as southern China and within Africa), there are low rates of DDH.

Increased Risk for DDH

Breech presentation at any time in pregnancy
Family history
Female
First born child
High birth weight/oligohydramnios
'Packaging disorders' (see text)

Symptoms/Signs

The signs present will depend on the age of the child being examined. The key for examination is to identify if the hip is dislocated, or if not, whether it is unstable.

In unilateral dislocation, asymmetrical reduction of hip abduction can be useful to identify abnormality, although this

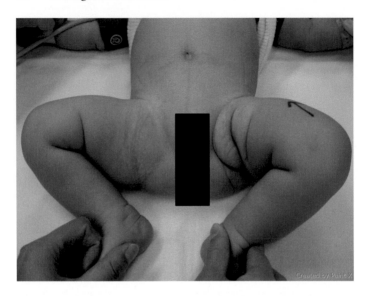

FIGURE 6.1 Photograph demonstrating asymmetry of thigh creases in left sided DDH

may be less helpful in the bilateral dislocation. Thigh skin crease asymmetry can be identified, although this is neither sensitive nor specific, with 1 in 4 children demonstrating some asymmetry (Fig. 6.1). Widening of the perineum may be noted on the affected side.

Leg lengths can be examined with the heels and knees together, looking for relative shortening of the femur (Galeazzi's test). This will demonstrate any cause for femoral shortening (e.g. proximal femoral focal deficiency) (see Chap. 13) and is not specific.

The widely used tests for screening in the neonate are the Barlow's and Ortolani's test. These tests are performed as part of a neonatal check and again at 6 weeks in the UK. The neonate is examined with the nappy removed, supine on a firm examination couch. The hips and knees are flexed to 90° and the hands placed over each thigh, with the middle finger

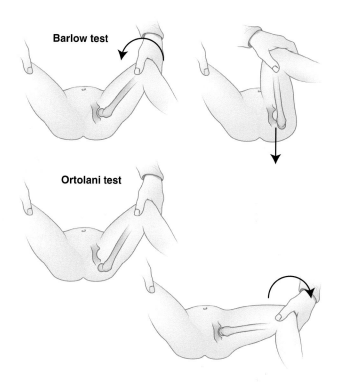

FIGURE 6.2 Diagram demonstrating the Barlow and Ortolani tests

resting on the greater trochanter and the thumb over the medial thigh.

Ortolani's test (Fig. 6.2) involves gentle abduction of both thighs combined with an elevation force applied by the middle finger on the greater trochanter. In the normal infant, full abduction to 90° should be achieved. If the hip is dislocated, then there will be reduced hip abduction and there may be a "clunk" of relocation as the femoral head relocates, moving over the posterior acetabular wall. If the hip is initially enlocated, or is dislocated and irreducible, this will not occur.

Barlow's test (Fig. 6.2) demonstrates instability of a reduced hip. With the hands in the same position as previously, the hips are held flexed to 90° and adducted. A posteriorly directed force is applied while feeling for the femoral head dislocating posteriorly with the middle fingers. Once again a "clunk" may be appreciated suggesting a dislocatable hip.

Both of these tests become less useful as the child grows older; by 3 months the increased muscle tone and stiffness prevent easy dislocation/relocation. For later diagnosis, the most sensitive test is measurement of abduction in 90° of flexion. The affected hip will demonstrate reduced abduction in comparison to the normal side.

In the walking child, a Trendelenburg gait may be observed, reflecting the defunctioning of the abductors. The child may walk on their tip-toes in view of the shortening on the affected side. The bilateral dislocation presenting at walking age demonstrates a "waddling" gait, often with an associated hyperlordosis of the lumbar spine.

Investigations

Imaging modality used is dependent on the age of the infant.

Ultrasound

Ultrasound is useful in the neonate with little ossification of the acetabulum and no ossification centre of the femoral head (<3 months). The use of ultrasound was initially introduced by Graf in the 1980s, using the method to classify the hip according to bony and cartilaginous morphology as viewed on a coronal section (Fig. 6.3a–d). The alpha angle is calculated according to the angle of coverage of the bony acetabular roof, the beta angle representing the cartilaginous roof and labrum. This method requires a reduced hip to produce accurate measurement (Table 6.1).

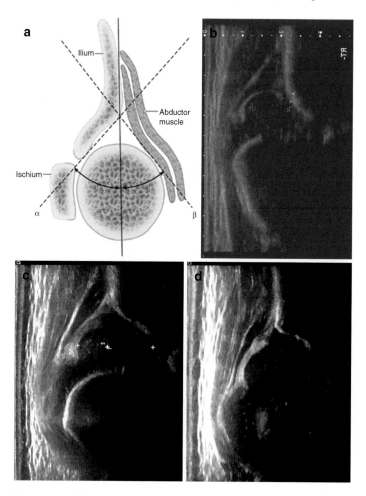

FIGURE 6.3 (a) Coronal section of hip demonstrating alpha and beta angles (reproduced with permission from *Tachdjian's Pediatric Orthopaedics*, ed 4. Philadelphia. WB Saunders). (b) Sonogram illustrating Graf IV (dislocated hip). (c) Sonogram illustrating a Graf IIc (alpha angle 48°) Hip at 6 weeks of age. Decision to treat with Pavlik Harness. (d) Sonogram of Hip (3c) after 6 weeks of Pavlik harness treatment, demonstrating normal acetabular morphology

TABLE 6.1 Sonographic classification according to Graf

Graf type	Alpha angle	Beta angle	Comment	Treatment
Ia	>60	<55	Normal hip	None
II*	50–59		Physiologically immature (<12 weeks)	Observation
IIa	50–59	<77	Shallow acetabulum (>12 weeks)	Pavlik Harness
IIb	50–59	<77	Delay of ossification of femoral head	Pavlik Harness
IIc	43–49	<77	Acetabular deficiency	Pavlik Harness
IId	43–49	>77	Everted cartilage roof/ labrum	Pavlik Harness
III	<43		Subluxed hip	Pavlik Harness
IV	Not measurable		Dislocated hip	Trial of reduction with Pavlik Harness

Dynamic methods have been demonstrated by Harcke, in which the Barlow and Ortolani tests are performed under ultrasound guidance. This provides information of stability, rather than morphology. The method is dependent on the skill and experience of the sonographer. Rosendahl described use of a combination of dynamic and static methods to allow the identification of both morphology and stability.

Plain Radiographs

Anteroposterior views of the pelvis and hips may be more useful from 3 months of age. Various lines have been

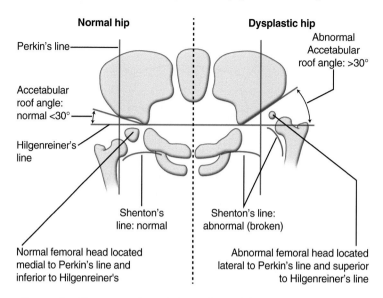

FIGURE 6.4 Demonstration of the radiographic parameters seen in the normal and dislocated hip

described to aid in the assessment of the paediatric radiograph (Fig. 6.4):

Shenton's line- A line following the medial neck of the femur should continue in an unbroken curve to follow the inferior edge of the pubis. This should be intact in any view of the pelvis; if disrupted then dislocation or subluxation should be suspected.

Hilgenreiner's and Perkin's lines – A straight horizontal line drawn between the triradiate cartilages in both hips. This can be used in conjunction with Perkin's line, which is a vertical line drawn down from the lateral edge of the acetabular sourcil, perpendicular to that of Hilgenreiner's line. The normal femoral head should lie in the inferior and medial quadrant produced by these two lines.

Acetabular index- the angle between Hilgenreiner's line and the slope of the acetabular sourcil forms the acetabular index. This should measure <30° at birth, falling to <20° by 2 years.

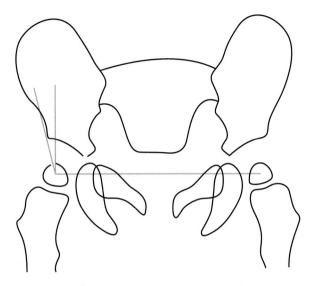

FIGURE 6.5 Lateral Centre edge angle of Wiburg (Reproduced with permission from Ozonoff MB: *Pediatric Orthopedic Radiology*. W.B. Saunders Company: Philadelphia, 1992)

Other measurable parameters include Sharp's Angle and the Centre edge angle of Wiberg (Fig. 6.5) Measurement of radiographic parameters in the child should be taken with caution. Inter and intraobserver variability has been noted for many of these measurements, not to mention the difficulty of accurately positioning the patient to prevent rotated images. The trend of measurements over time is more valuable than the measurements made on a singe radiograph.

Treatment

The goal of treatment is to ensure the femoral head is reduced within the acetabulum in a stable and concentric manner, to allow normal development of the joint. The modality of treatment used is guided primarily on the age of

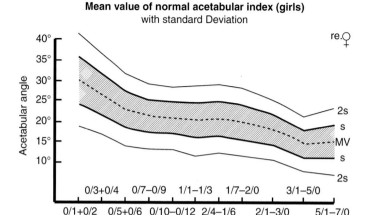

FIGURE 6.6 Graph demonstrating mean value of acetabular index in girls (reproduced with permission from Tonnis D. Normal values of the hip joint for the evaluation of X-rays in children and adults. *Clinical orthopaedics and related research*. 1976:39–47.)

the patient at the time of diagnosis. The greatest period of acetabular remodelling is in the first 3–6 months of age, so earlier treatment is preferred (Fig. 6.6).

The infant who has instability on postnatal screening with evidence of dysplasia on ultrasound, but a concentrically reduced hip (Graf II), may be initially treated with observation and serial examination as spontaneous improvement may be seen in the first 6 weeks. If no improvement, with ongoing evidence of instability, or deterioration is seen over this period, then splinting should be considered.

In the presence of more significant dysplasia with subluxation or dislocation (Graf III/IV) splinting may be considered from the initial consultation. A number of devices have been described (Pavlik harness, Von Rosen splint, Frejka Pillow) each of which aim to hold the hip in a position of abduction and flexion, to encourage a concentric reduction of the hip joint. The most commonly used device is the Pavlik harness (Fig. 6.7).

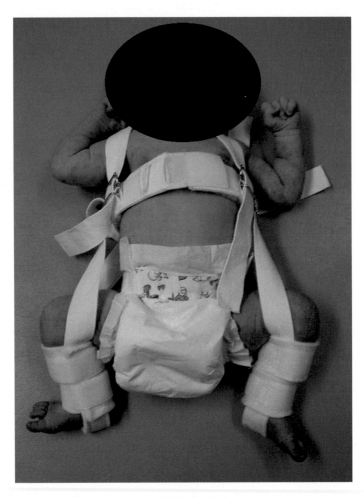

FIGURE 6.7 Photograph of child in Pavlik harness

Pavlik Harness

The use of Pavlik harness depends on whether it is to guide the reduction of a dislocated hip or to maintain reduction of a reduced/dislocatable hip. To guide reduction, the hip is held in 90° of flexion with abduction to aim the metaphysis of the proximal femur towards the triradiate cartilage. For the dislocated, irreducible hip, the harness can be trialled with careful monitoring. If reduction is not achieved within the first 2 weeks, then splinting should be abandoned to avoid risks of complications associated with pressure on the femoral head and posterior acetabular wall.

Once reduction is achieved, the aim of the prosthesis is to prevent the leg moving into the unstable position of extension and abduction, while allowing some movement of further abduction/flexion. The legs should be positioned in approximately 100–110° of flexion. Forced abduction should be avoided with the aim to position the leg in the "safe zone" between unforced abduction and the degree of ab/adduction where the hip redislocates. The child is monitored every 2 weeks to ensure correct positioning of the brace and ensure concentric reduction is maintained. Adjustment of the brace and /or straps are required as the child grows to prevent the legs being held in excessive flexion or abduction. Following concentric reduction of the hip, the brace is continued until the alpha angle >60 deg and the hip is stable.

In the infant under 3 months of age, a 95% success rate has been described in the unstable hip. In the dislocated hip the success rate is approximately 85%. The rates of success decrease with increasing age to 50% in the 6 month old, partly reflecting the difficulty in maintaining bracing in the more active and mobile child. Failure rates would be expected to be higher in patients where there is a teratological cause for dislocation, such as arthrogryposis or myelomeningocoele.

Possible complications relating to the Pavlik harness mainly relate to improper positioning of the orthosis, but include:

- Skin irritation, if scrupulous hygiene is not maintained.
- Brachial plexus injury, due to excessive tightening of the shoulder straps.
- Femoral nerve palsy if a hyperflexed position is maintained.
- Damage to the femoral head or proximal physis. This is the most significant of complications, associated with excessive abduction or continued treatment despite failure of reduction of the head.

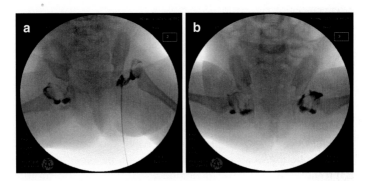

FIGURE 6.8 (**a**) Arthrogram demonstrating left sided dislocated hip prior to closed reduction. (**b**) Arthrogram demonstrating enlocated left hip following closed reduction

- "Pavlik harness disease", which is caused by prolonged use of the harness with the irreducible hip in a dislocated position. The resulting posterior acetabular deficiency can increase the risk of failure of a later closed reduction and may necessitate further pelvic osteotomies to manage the posterior instability.

Closed Reduction

If the Pavlik harness treatment fails, is not suitable or the child presents >6 months of age, then a formal closed reduction can be performed under a general anaesthetic. An arthrogram is performed as an initial step (Fig. 6.8a–b). This allows clear demonstration of the position of the cartilaginous component of the femoral head and acetabulum as well as potential blocks to reduction. Dynamic screening can allow demonstration of the reduction and the position of stability to maintain this reduction. If there is a narrow safe zone between unforced abduction and redislocation, secondary to an adduction contracture, then a percutaneous adductor tenotomy is performed. This allows a greater arc of unforced abduction and aims to reduce the pressure on the

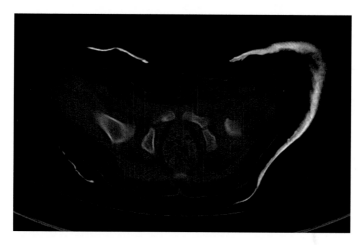

FIGURE 6.9 Axial CT image demonstrating of plaster moulding around greater trochanters

femoral head. Psoas tenotomy can also be performed if required to maintain a stable reduction.

Following reduction, the child is placed in a bilateral below knee hip spica with the hip flexed to 90° and held in the safe zone of abduction. Careful moulding of the plaster is required around the greater trochanters to ensure that the reduction is maintained. The spica is continued for 12 weeks with a review at 6 weeks to ensure that reduction is maintained. This can be performed with either plain radiographs, or less commonly with a short segment CT (Fig. 6.9).

Open Reduction

If a closed reduction fails, cannot be achieved, or if forced abduction is required to maintain reduction, then the closed reduction should be abandoned for an open procedure. Open reduction of the hip should aim to address the structures, which block the reduction of the femoral head (Red box 2). This procedure can be performed through a medial or more commonly, an anterior approach, the latter less likely to lead to avascular necrosis as a complication.

Blocks to reduction of the femoral head

Intra-articular
- Hypertrophied ligamentum teres.
- Pulvinar.
- Shortened/thickened transverse acetabular ligament.

Extra-articular
- Iliopsoas tendon (hourglass constriction of capsule on arthrogram).
- Adductor longus.

Following reduction, a test of stability is performed to assess the requirement for further osteotomies; the stability of the hip is dependent on the depth and quality of the acetabulum. This should be performed prior to any capsular plication. A hip spica is applied below the knee on the operated side, above the knee on the contralateral side. Immobilisation is maintained for 12 weeks.

Osteotomies

The decision making process for the requirement of osteotomies depends on a number of factors (Fig. 6.10, Table 6.2):

- Stability.
- Age of the patient at the time of reduction – the younger the patient, the greater the remodelling potential.
- Radiographic parameters – can identify risk of poor progression and potential for residual dysplasia.

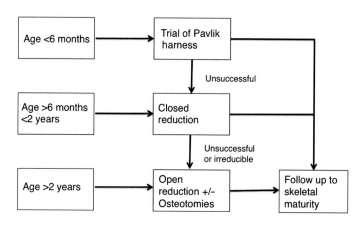

FIGURE 6.10 Flow chart demonstrating treatment options at different ages of presentation

There are various types of osteotomies that can be used. These include:

Pelvic osteotomies

The aim is to improve the coverage of the femoral head. There are a variety of different techniques described, which can be divided into three main groups: rotational/redirectional, volume reducing and salvage osteotomies.

- *Redirectional osteotomies* – This group aims to correct coverage of the femoral head. A congruent hip is required for this procedure to be successful. Examples include Dega and Salter osteotomies.
- *Volume reducing osteotomies* – An anterolateral wall defect can lead to a "double diameter" acetabulum, in which a congruent fit cannot be achieved due to a mismatch between the femoral head size and that of the larger acetabulum. In this situation a volume reducing osteotomy may be utilised to achieve anterolateral coverage and a congruent joint. An example is a Pemberton osteotomy.

TABLE 6.2 Decision planning algorithm for osteotomies

Femoral osteotomy indications		Pelvic osteotomy indications	
Reduction only stable with A. Int Rotation B. Abduction C. Int & Abduction	Excess soft tissue tension despite release	Normal size acetabulum, concentric reduction, acetabular dysplasia secondary to acetabular mal-orientation	Concentric reduction not possible
Treatment		**Treatment**	
A. Derotation osteotomy B. Varus osteotomy C. Varus and Derotation	Femoral Shortening ± Column 1	Dega or Salter Osteotomy (age 18 m – 8 years) Triple Pelvic Osteotomy (6 years to skeletal maturity) Peri-acetabular osteotomy (after skeletal maturity)	Large acetabulum (Pemberton if deficient anterior coverage) Dega also useful for efficient posterior coverage. Small acetabulum (Shelf or Chiari Osteotomy)
If acetabular dysplasia present assess for Pelvic Osteotomy			

- *Salvage Osteotomy* – In situations where adequate coverage or concentric reduction is not achievable, a salvage procedure can be used, often in older children. The aim of these procedures is to provide coverage of the proximal femur with fibrocartilaginous metaplasia, rather than the hyaline cartilage of the acetabulum. Examples include Shelf, and less commonly, Chiari, osteotomies.

Proximal femoral osteotomies

In the patient requiring excessive tension to maintain reduction of the hip, a shortening femoral osteotomy may be used. Shortening is often required in reduction of the established dislocated hip to reduce the pressure applied to the femoral head and as such the risk of avascular necrosis and growth disturbance. In the older child with closure of the triradiate cartilage, a proximal femoral osteotomy alone will not improve the dysplasia of the acetabular side, as the remodelling potential has been lost. If combined with an acetabular redirectional osteotomy, the risk of overcorrection arises, with possible posterior instability.

Complications

Avascular necrosis (AVN) of the proximal femur is a sequela of intervention in DDH; it is not seen in the untreated patient. Forced abduction splintage, tight reduction or direct vascular injury at the time of surgery may be the implicated. Some degree of AVN is frequently observed; however it is the severity of the disturbance, which is important. Damage to the physis can result in growth disturbance or arrest and femoral head deformities, with secondary acetabular changes. These changes may only become apparent in the adolescent growth spurt.

Other complications include redislocation and neurovascular injury.

Follow-Up

Follow-up of treated patients should continue until skeletal maturity. At this point, Murphy et al. have demonstrated that an acetabular index of >15° or a lateral centre edge angle of greater than 16° is associated with an early onset of osteoarthritis. However, there is great debate as to the correct threshold for performing secondary procedures, depending on the degree of expected remodelling remaining. Different studies have estimated the period of remodelling potential to be as low as 2 years or up to 11 years, although it likely lies between the two.

At each review, the radiographs should demonstrate a congruent hip with maintained Shenton's line, an improvement in the acetabular index and any evidence of AVN should be noted. Identification of complications of AVN and residual dysplasia is required to allow timely correction with further bony procedures. Taking the upper threshold of acetabular index of 28° at 4 years following reduction may result in the lowest level of false positive rates for the requirement of further procedures.

Criteria for assessment at each follow up in clinic

Clinical
- Assess range of motion.
- Leg length discrepancy.

Radiographic - on AP pelvis
- Assess Shenton's line.
- Measure acetabular index, centre-edge angle.
- Look for evidence of AVN.

Classification Systems

- Severin classification for radiographic outcomes after treatment (Table 6.3).
- Bucholz-Ogden Classification for AVN of the proximal femur (Table 6.4).

TABLE 6.3 Severin classification for radiographic outcomes after treatment

Group	Criteria
I	Normal hip
II	Concentric reduction of the joint with moderate deformity of the femoral neck, head or acetabulum
III	Dysplasia but no subluxation
IV	Subluxation
V	Articulation with false acetabulum relating to original acetabulum
VI	Redislocation

TABLE 6.4 Bucholz-Ogden classification for AVN of the proximal femur

Grade	Area involved	Effect
I	Changes limited to proximal femoral epiphysis	Hypoplastic epiphysis, no significant growth disturbance
II	Lateral physeal and metaphyseal damage and tethering	Valgus femoral neck deformity
III	Entire physis and metaphysis involved	Coxa breva with trochanteric overgrowth. Asphericity of femoral head
IV	Medial physeal and metaphyseal injury	Varus femoral neck deformity

Synopsis

Developmental dysplasia of the hip represents a spectrum of deformity. The aim of treatment is to obtain a stable and congruent hip in order to allow comfortable ambulation and postpone the onset of osteoarthritis. Early detection and management is important as later diagnosis will often require a more aggressive intervention and be associated with a poorer final outcome result.

Key References

Barlow TG. Early diagnosis and treatment of congenital dislocation of the hip. J Bone Joint Surg Br. 1962;44-B(2):292–301.

Cashman JP, Round J, Taylor G, et al. The natural history of developmental dysplasia of the hip after early supervised treatment in the Pavlik harness. A prospective, longitudinal follow up. J Bone Joint Surg Br. 2002;84(3):418–25.

Zadeh HG, Catterall A, Hashemi-Nejad A, Perry RE. Test of stability as an aid to decide the need for osteotomy in association with open reduction in developmental dysplasia of the hip. J Bone Joint Surg Br. 2000;82(1):17–27.

Albinana J, Dolan L, Spratt K, et al. Acetabular dysplasia after treatment for developmental dysplasia of the hip. Implications for secondary procedures. J Bone Joint Surg. 2004;86B:876–86.

Murphy SB, Ganz R, Muller ME. The prognosis in untreated dysplasia of the hip. A study of radiographic factors that predict the outcome. J Bone Joint Surg Am. 1995;77:985–9.

Chapter 7
Legg-Calvé-Perthes' Disease

Daud Tai Shan Chou and Manoj Ramachandran

Introduction

Legg-Calvé-Perthes' disease (LCPD) is an idiopathic childhood hip disorder that produces ischaemic necrosis of the growing femoral head. Subchondral stress fractures of the necrotic bone initiate a pathological repair process with an imbalance between bone resorption and formation. The new bone formed results in a flattened and enlarged femoral head, which gradually remodels until skeletal maturity.

Epidemiology

LCPD is a rare disease that affects boys four to five times more than girls. The peak incidence is between the ages of 4 and 8, although LCPD has been reported in patients as young

D.T.S. Chou, MBBS, BSc, MRCS (Tr&Orth)
T&O SpR Percivall Pott Rotation, London, UK

M. Ramachandran, BSc, MBBS, FRCS (T&O) (✉)
Paediatric and Young Adult Orthopaedic Unit,
The Royal London and Barts and The London Children's
Hospitals, Barts Health, London, UK
e-mail: manojorthopod@gmail.com

N.A. Aresti et al. (eds.), *Paediatric Orthopaedics
in Clinical Practice*, In Clinical Practice,
DOI 10.1007/978-1-4471-6769-3_7,
© Springer-Verlag London 2016

as 2 and as old as 13. Many children are generally shorter than average and have delayed bone ages compared to their chronological age. This usually returns to normal after healing of the disease. Bilateral involvement is seen in about 10% of cases and the two femoral heads, at diagnosis, are usually at different stages of collapse.

Aetiology

LCPD is initiated by avascular necrosis of the femoral head; however the cause of this impairment of blood supply is still unknown.

Current theories include:

- Trauma.
- Infection.
- Endocrine/metabolic disorders.
- Genetic – missense mutation in type II collagen gene.
- Thrombosis or venous obstruction.

Pathogenesis

Histopathological studies of the femoral head in LCPD have shown a number of changes, described below, which have formed the basis of our current understanding of the disease pathogenesis (Table 7.1). In principle, ischaemia produces a decrease in mechanical strength of the femoral head resulting in accumulation of microfractures in the necrotic bone. Vascular invasion and resorption further compromise the mechanical strength of the femoral head leading to femoral head deformity.

Symptoms/Signs

The majority of patients present with mild hip pain of insidious onset, a limp and/or reduced hip movements. Pain is usually activity related and localised to the groin but can be referred to the thigh and knee area.

TABLE 7.1 Pathological processes in LCPD

	Initial stage	Resorption stage	Reparative stage
Articular cartilage	Necrosis in deep layer Cessation of endochondral ossification Separation from underlying subchondral bone	Vascular invasion New accessory ossification	Irregularly hypertrophied articular cartilage
Bony epiphysis	Necrosis of marrow space and trabecular bone	Invasion of vascular connective tissue Compression fracture of trabeculae Osteoclastic resorption of necrotic bone	Assymetric appearance of normal bone
Physis	Irregularity in the columnisation of cartilaginous growth cells	May extend inferiorly	Growth disturbance apparent
Metaphysis	Fibrocartilage Fat necrosis	Vascular proliferation Disorganised ossification	

On examination, an antalgic or Trendelenburg gait may be observed. Hip motion is usually maintained at the early stages but both synovitis and abductor spasm may result in some hip irritability. Initially, hip internal rotation and abduction are limited followed by limitation of other hip movements. During the fragmentation stage, hip motion can become severely restricted with the development of flexion and abduction contractures in some patients. Atrophy of the thigh and calf muscles may be present from disuse, secondary to pain. There may be a leg length discrepancy either from true shortening at the collapsed femoral epiphysis or apparent shortening due to an abduction contracture.

Investigations

The primary imaging modality for LCPD is plain radiographs; standing anteroposterior and frog-leg lateral views of both hips. These X-rays aid in initial diagnosis, staging of the disease and in providing information about the prognosis.

Additional imaging studies to consider:

- Bone scanning may reveal the avascularity of the femoral head in the early stages of the disease.
- MRI can detect changes in bone perfusion when X-ray changes are not apparent. However the clinical and prognostic relevance of MRI has yet to be formally defined in the management of LCPD.
- Arthrography is useful to assess the shape of the femoral head in relation to the acetabulum and is used to plan surgical management.

Radiographic Stages

LCDP has been divided into four radiographic stages according to characteristic features initially described by Waldenstrom:

1. Initial Stage:
   - Lateralisation of the femoral head.
   - Decreased size of the ossification centre.
   - Subchondral fracture.
   - Metaphyseal lucencies.

2. Fragmentation Stage:

- Fragmented epiphyses.
- Areas of radiolucency and radiodensity.
- This stage lasts about 1 year.

3. Re-ossification (Healing) Stage:

- Bone density returns to normal.
- This stage usually lasts 3–5 years.

4. Residual (Healed) Stage:

- Femoral head fully re-ossified.
- Remodelling of the head and acetabulum until skeletal maturity.

Classification Systems

Four different classification systems have been described:

Catterall

Based on the amount of capital femoral epiphysis (CFE) involvement on X-rays taken at the fragmentation stage of the disease

Group I – Anterior CFE involvement only
Group II – up to 50% involvement with metaphyseal cysts
Group III – up to 75% involvement with large sequestrum
Group IV – The whole of femoral head involved

Stulberg Outcome Classification

Stulberg outcome classification is determined using both AP and frog lateral radiographs at skeletal maturity (Table 7.2).

TABLE 7.2 Stulberg classification summary

Class	Indications	Prognosis
I – Spherical congruency	Completely normal hip joint	Good

II – Spherical congruency with less than 2 mm loss of head shape	Spherical femoral head with a concentric circle on radiographs, with 1 or more of the following abnormalities:
	    Coxa magna
	    Short femoral neck
	    Abnormally steep acetabulum
		Good

III – Aspherical congruency with greater than 2 mm loss of head shape	Non-spherical (ovoid/mushroom shaped), but not a flat femoral head. With class II characteristics	Mild to moderate osteoarthritis
IV – Aspherical congruency	Flat femoral head with abnormalities of the femoral head, neck and acetabulum	Mild to moderate osteoarthritis
V – Aspherical incongruency	Flat femoral head with a normal neck and acetabulum	Severe and early osteoarthritis

Salter-Thompson Classification

This classification system is determined on X-rays during the early phase of the disease. It is based on the extent and location of subchondral fracture of the femoral head, which relates to the amount of subsequent bone resorption.

Group A – Less than 50% of the femoral head involved
Group B – More than 50% of the femoral head involved

Herring Lateral Pillar Classification (Modified in 2004)

This is determined on an AP hip X-ray in the early fragmentation stage of the disease. A radiolucent line of fragmentation separates the lateral pillar from the central portion of the femoral head or the lateral quarter of the femoral head represents the lateral pillar (Fig. 7.1).

Group A (Fig. 7.2) – No loss of density or height of the lateral pillar

Group B (Fig. 7.3) – Lucency in the lateral pillar and <50% loss of height

Group B/C border
- Exactly 50% loss of lateral pillar height.
- <50% loss of height but with a very narrow lateral pillar or very little ossification of the lateral pillar.

Group C (Fig. 7.4) – Lucency in the lateral pillar and >50% loss of height

The Herring lateral pillar classification system has been shown to have better interobserver reliability than the

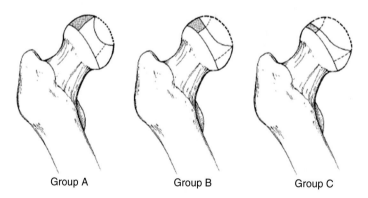

Group A   Group B   Group C

FIGURE 7.1 Herring Lateral Pillar classification system (Reproduced with permission from Skaggs and Tolo)

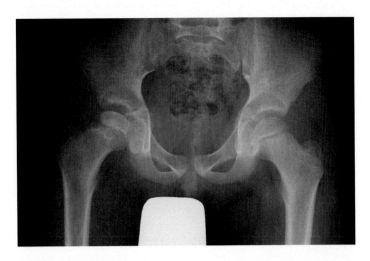

FIGURE 7.2 Herring A

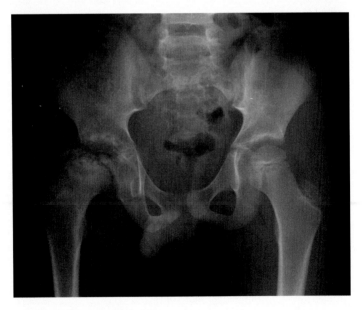

FIGURE 7.3 Herring B

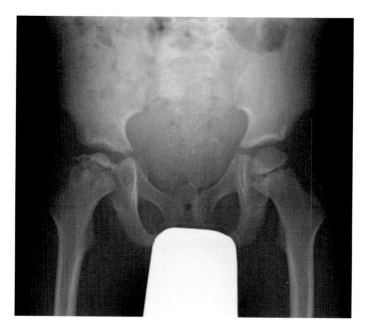

FIGURE 7.4 Herring C

Catterall classification. It has often been used to provide prognostic information and guide management.

Prognostic Factors

Various clinical and radiographic features have been identified as prognostic indicators of outcome.

- Age at onset – good prognosis if onset <5; poor if onset >9; due to the tri-radiate cartilage fusing at the age of 8.
- Catterral classification and four radiographic head at-risk signs:
    - Gage sign – radiolucency of the lateral epiphysis and metaphysis.
    - Lateral calcification.

  – Lateral capital femoral epiphysis subluxation.
  – Horizontal physis.

- Premature physeal closure.
- Lateral pillar height at fragmentation stage – Herring lateral pillar classification.
- Extent of subchondral fracture – Salter-Thompson classification.
- Extent of femoral head deformity and loss of hip joint congruity at maturity – Stulberg classification.
- Extent of femoral head deformity as early marker of prognosis – deformity index.

Differential Diagnosis

In the early phase of the disease the diagnosis of LCPD must be differentiated from septic arthritis with or without osteomyelitis of the proximal femur.

The differential diagnosis of LCPD includes:

- Reactive synovitis.
- Septic arthritis.
- Osteomyelitis of the proximal femur.
- Juvenile arthritis.
- Osteonecrosis of the femoral head, due to one of the following:

  – Sickle cell anaemia.
  – Thalassaemia.
  – Haemophilia.
  – Idiopathic thrombocytopaenia purpura.
  – Leukaemia.
  – Gaucher's disease.

In bilateral cases the differential diagnosis becomes more difficult. However, it is worth remembering that bilateral LCPD is virtually never simultaneous. Diagnoses to consider in the case of bilateral signs, would include:

- Skeletal dysplasia e.g. multiple epiphyseal dysplasia.
- Hypothyroidism.
- Genetic syndromes e.g. trichorhinophalangeal syndrome.

Treatment

The main goals of treatment in LCPD are to relieve symptoms, preserve the sphericity of the femoral head, maintain normal hip range of motion and to prevent degenerative arthritis.

- Symptomatic treatment:

  - Non-steroidal anti-inflammatory drugs.
  - Short periods of protected weight bearing with crutches.
  - Bed rest and traction.

- Non-surgical containment:

  - Activity restriction (e.g. running and jumping).
  - Orthotic devices, e.g. Petrie abduction cast, A-frame or Atlanta Scottish Rite orthosis. No standardised treatment protocol exists for orthotic devices, but in principle, abduction devices should be continued until subchondral re-ossification is demonstrated. Only retrospective studies have shown the effectiveness of these treatments and they are less frequently used in contemporary treatment regimens.

- Surgical containment:

  - Proximal femoral varus osteotomy.

    - Effective in the early and fragmentation stage of the disease.
    - Performed when there is flattening or incongruity of the femoral head.
    - There is a risk of persistent varus angulation, trochanteric prominence and leg length discrepancy.

  - Reconstructive pelvic osteotomy e.g. Salter, Dega.

    - Best performed early in the disease and not during the remodelling stage.

- • Requires the femoral head to be almost round and the joint congruency demonstrated on hip arthrography.
  - • Rotation of the acetabulum should achieve anterior and lateral cover of the femoral head.
- – Acetabular shelf osteotomy (Fig. 7.5) (labral support procedure).

  - • Autologous iliac crest bone graft is used to achieve an extension of the acetabulum, thus preventing sub-luxation and lateral overgrowth of the epiphysis.
  - • After the procedure, either an abduction brace or no bracing is preferable to a hip spica cast, to avoid a significant flexion contracture.

- – Combined pelvic and femoral procedures.

  - • Theoretical advantages include better femoral head containment without the complications of over-correcting if either procedure was performed alone.

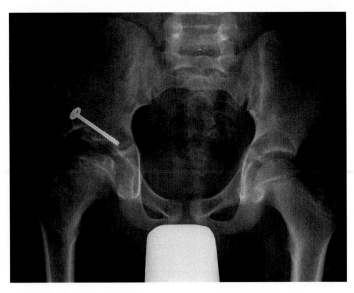

FIGURE 7.5 Shelf osteotomy for containment

- Late surgery for deformity.

  - Chiari osteotomy (medial displacement osteotomy) – when the femoral head is no longer containable.
  - Acetabular shelf osteotomy (labral support procedure) – application of bone graft to lateral aspect of acetabulum to cover uncontained femoral head.
  - Cheilectomy – partial capital resection for a deformed head or hinge abduction.
  - Abduction extension osteotomy – for hinge abduction.

- Late surgery for osteoarthritis.

  - Total hip replacement.

The exact management of LCPD remains controversial; however it is important to understand the general principles that should guide treatment. The concept of containment is based on preventing deformity of the femoral head by maintaining the head within the depth of the acetabulum thereby equalising the pressure and subjecting it to the moulding action of the acetabulum.

Treatment should be guided by age of disease onset, prognostic factors and current best evidence.

- Age of onset <6–8 years

  - Treat symptomatically.

- Age of onset >6–8 years

  - Initially treat symptomatically until Herring classification has been determined.
  - Herring A, C – treat non-operatively.
  - Herring B, B/C – treat operatively to achieve containment).

Deformities at Maturity (Fig. 7.6)

- Coxa magna – enlarged head.
- Coxa brevis – short neck and overgrowth of greater trochanter as a result of premature femoral neck physeal growth arrest.

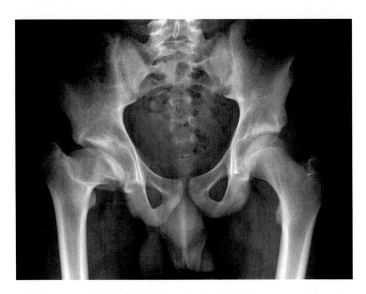

FIGURE 7.6 Residual deformity – trochanteric overgrowth, coxa magna and coxa breva

- Hinge abduction – Acetabular rim impingement against enlarged laterally extruded femoral head when the hip is abducted.
- Osteochondritis dissecans.

Synopsis

LCPD is an idiopathic avascular necrosis of the femoral head characterised by hip pain or reduced hip movements in children aged between 4 and 8. Plain AP and lateral radiographs are usually sufficient to make the diagnosis. Although the management of LCPD is controversial the main goals of treatment are to retain femoral head sphericity and maintain hip range of motion. Prognosis depends on the age of onset and the extent of femoral head involvement.

Historical Note

In 1910, coxa plana was independently described by Arthur Legg in the United States, Jacques Calvé in France and George Perthes in Germany. Henning Waldenström gave an accurate description of the disease in 1909, but he believed that it was a benign form of tuberculosis. Although many credit the first description of Perthes' disease to Waldenström, it was Austrian surgeon Karel Maydl (1853–1903) who first published on the topic in 1897.

Key References

Aresti N, Ramachandran M. Nonoriginal Malappropriate Eponymous Nomenclature: examples relevant to paediatric orthopaedics. J Pediatr Orthop B. 2012;21(6):606–10.

Catterall A. The natural history of Perthes' disease. J Bone Joint Surg Br. 1971;53(1):37–53.

Stulberg SD, Cooperman DR, Wallensten R. The natural history of Legg-Calve-Perthes disease. J Bone Joint Surg Am. 1981;63(7): 1095–108.

Salter RB, Thompson GH. Legg-Calve-Perthes disease. The prognostic significance of the subchondral fracture and a two-group classification of the femoral head involvement. J Bone Joint Surg Am. 1984;66(4):479–89.

Herring JA, et al. The lateral pillar classification of Legg-Calve-Perthes disease. J Pediatr Orthop. 1992;12(2):143–50.

Herring JA, Kim HT, Browne R. Legg-Calve-Perthes disease. Part I: classification of radiographs with use of the modified lateral pillar and Stulberg classifications. J Bone Joint Surg Am. 2004;86-A(10): 2103–20.

Skaggs DL, Tolo VT. Legg-Calve-Perthes disease. J Am Acad Orthop Surg. 1996;4(1):9–16.

Chapter 8
Slipped Capital Femoral Epiphysis

Lucky Jeyaseelan and Kyle James

Introduction

Slipped capital femoral epiphysis (SCFE) or slipped femoral capital epiphysis (SUFE) occurs following failure of the proximal femoral physis, resulting in displacement of the proximal femoral epiphysis relative to the femoral neck and shaft (Fig. 8.1). The displacement of the physis is referred to as posterior and medial. However, the epiphysis actually remains within the acetabulum and it is the neck and shaft that displace anteriorly and externally rotate.

L. Jeyaseelan, MBBS, BSc (Hons), MRCS
T&O SpR Percivall Pott Rotation, London, UK

K. James, FRCS (Tr&Orth) (✉)
Paediatric and Young Adult Orthopaedic Unit,
The Royal London and Barts and The London Children's
Hospitals, Barts Health, London, UK
e-mail: Kyle.James@bartshealth.nhs.uk

N.A. Aresti et al. (eds.), *Paediatric Orthopaedics in Clinical Practice*, In Clinical Practice, DOI 10.1007/978-1-4471-6769-3_8, © Springer-Verlag London 2016

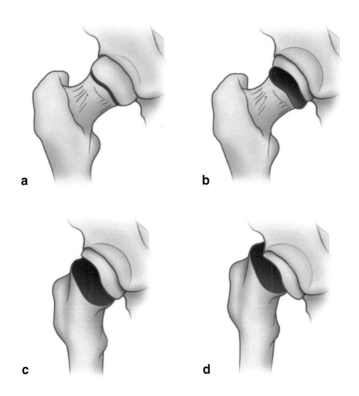

FIGURE 8.1 Diagram demonstrating the displacement of the proximal femoral epiphysis and subsequent rotation of the femoral neck relative to the head. (**a**) Normal, (**b**) mild, (**c**) moderate, and (**d**) severe

Epidemiology

SCFE is the most frequent hip disorder amongst adolescents and occurs during the adolescent growth spurt. Males are more commonly affected than females by a ratio of 3.2:1 Incidence rates are between 2 and 10 in 100,000. At time of presentation, most boys are aged between 12 and 15 years and most girls between 10 and 13 years. Obesity is a well-defined feature of SCFE with over half of affected children weighing over the 95 centile for their age group. There are significant differences in incidence among differing races, with African Americans and Polynesians having the highest rates.

In unilateral cases, the left hip is more commonly affected. Up to 20% of cases will be bilateral at presentation. Of the 80% unilateral cases, 20–40% will develop a symptomatic slip of the contralateral side during adolescence, the majority if these occurring within 18 months from diagnosis of the initial slip.

Aetiology

The exact aetiology of SCFE is unclear. Local anatomical and perhaps hormonal changes cause mechanical instability of the proximal femoral physis with inability to resist load across it. The failure of the physis across the hypertrophic zone results in the slippage.

There are numerous conditions associated with SCFE and the susceptible physis. These include:

- Endocrine factors:

  - The most common endocrine conditions in children with SCFE are:

    - Hypothyroidism.
    - Panhypopituitarism.
    - Growth hormone abnormalities.
    - Hypogonadism.

  - Other endocrine causes include:

    - Hyperparathyroidism.
    - Renal osteodystrophy.

      - Up to eightfold increase in risk for SUFE.
      - Due to secondary hyperparathyroidism.

- Mechanical factors.

  - Femoral neck retroversion.
  - Decreased femoral neck-shaft angle.
  - Superior acetabular retroversion and increased superolateral femoral head coverage.
  - Increased acetabular depth.

- Syndromic factors.

  - Trisomy 21 (Down's syndrome).

Pathogenesis

Histological analyses of the physis in SCFE suggest general disorganisation of the growth plate, with increased chrondroblast cell turnover (apoptosis). There is clear abnormality within the hypertrophic zone, which is found to be wider than the resting zone, with a reduced amount of collagen with poor orientation and poor columnar organisation of the cells.

Symptoms and Signs

Onset of symptoms may be sudden or, more commonly, gradually develop over the preceding weeks or months. Typically, the patient will complain of pain in the hip or groin. Thigh pain is also a common symptom and up to 25% of children may present with knee pain.

On examination, the child may walk with an antalgic or Trendelenburg gait, with the affected limb in external rotation. There is increasing limitation of hip movements with increasing severity of SCFE. Obligatory external rotation on passive hip flexion (Drennan's sign), with an associated loss of internal rotation is a common finding. Limb shortening is seen in severe cases. Patients with an unstable slip demonstrate complete inability to bear weight even with support and often are reluctant to move the limb.

> Weight bearing is the most important feature of a SCFE. Inability to weight bear suggests the patient has an unstable slip.

Investigations

Plain radiographs of both hips are the standard imaging modality in SCFE. Anteroposterior (AP) and lateral radiographs are sufficient to confirm the diagnosis. The earliest findings can be seen on lateral radiographs.

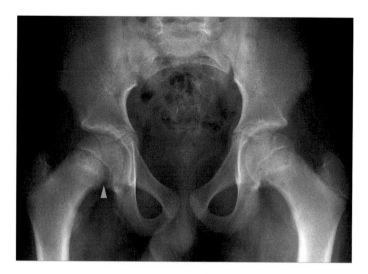

FIGURE 8.2 AP radiograph showing Klein's line and the metaphyseal blanch sign, *arrowhead*

Radiographic features on AP (Fig. 8.2) or shoot through/frog lateral (Fig. 8.4) radiographs include:

1. Widening and irregularity of the physis.
2. Decreased height of the capital femoral epiphysis (seen when the epiphysis lies behind the femoral neck).
3. Metaphyseal blanch sign – a dense crescent shaped area caused by the superimposed displaced epiphysis (arrow Fig. 8.2).
4. Callus formation in chronic slips.
5. Part of the femoral epiphysis normally lies lateral to Klein's line, a line drawn along the lateral aspect of the femoral neck. In SCFE, the line does not pass through the femoral head; this is known as Trethowan's sign. Comparison with the contralateral side may be useful (Figs. 8.2 and 8.3).

Features on lateral radiographs include:

1. Posterior step off and slipping of the epiphysis, or posterior callus (Fig. 8.4).
2. Southwick angle (Fig. 8.5).

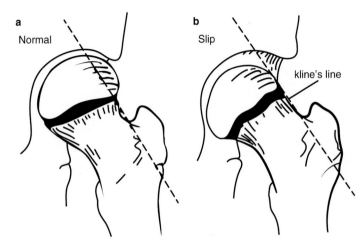

FIGURE 8.3 (**a**, **b**) Klein's line in (**a**) normal and (**b**) SCFE (Reproduced from Houghton, KM, Review for the generalist: evaluation of pediatric hip pain, *Pediatric Rheumatology*, 2009 7:10)

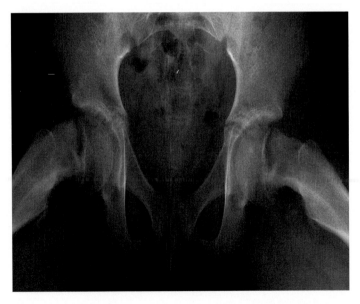

FIGURE 8.4 Frog leg lateral radiograph of a bilateral SCFE

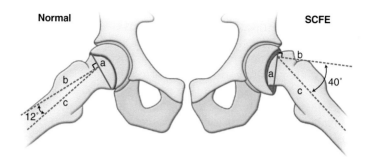

FIGURE 8.5 Diagrammatic representation of the Southwick angle. *a* Line connecting anterior and posterior margins of the physis, *b* line perpendicular to *a*, *c* line marking the centre of femoral neck and shaft

- The epiphyseal-shaft angle of the affected side subtracted from the normal side.
- The normal epiphyseal shaft angle is around 10–12°.

Computed tomography (CT) has limited benefit in SCFE. Situations where it is useful, includes:

- In late presentations of SUFE, to assess the degree of physeal closure. If closed, correction can generally only be safely achieved with extracapsular osteotomies in order to avoid avascular necrosis.
- In the presence of femoral head collapse, secondary to avascular necrosis, to assess penetration of metalwork in to the joint.

Magnetic resonance imaging (MRI) plays a specific role in those children in whom a diagnosis of SCFE is highly suspected but who have normal plain radiographs. MRI findings include:

1. Physeal widening.
2. Physeal irregularity.
3. Bone oedema adjacent to the physis.

All these aforementioned MRI findings are associated with a pre-slip state. Perfusion MRI scans can also be used to assess femoral head vascularity preoperatively in unstable slips where osteonecrosis is a concern. Post-operative use of MRI is often limited due to metal artefact.

SPECT and SPECT-CT play a specific role in post-operative assessment of femoral head vascularity and is a novel and probably reliable predictor of avascular necrosis.

Classifications

Numerous classifications systems for SCFE have been described.

Traditionally, SCFE was classified based on the duration of symptoms with no consideration for the stability of the slip, namely:

Pre-slip	Radiographic findings of irregularity, widening and fuzziness of the physis
Acute	Sudden onset, duration of symptoms less than 3 weeks
Chronic	Symptoms for more than 3 weeks
Acute-on-Chronic	Symptoms for more than 3 weeks with an acute exacerbation of pain

The Loder Classification is perhaps the most commonly now used. It considers the stability of the slip and is outcome related with predictability of avascular necrosis.

Stable slip	The child can weight bear with or without crutches
	Minimal risk of AVN (<1%)
Unstable slip	The child cannot weight bear at all
	High risk of AVN (between 10 and 60%)

Wilson described a classification based on the severity of the slip:

Grade I – 0–33% of the metaphysis is uncovered – mild slip.
Grade II – 33–50% uncovered – moderate slip.
Grade III – >50% uncovered – severe slip.

Carney's Classification is based on the Southwick angle, which is described above and illustrated in Fig. 8.5.

Grade I: mild <30°.
Grade II: moderate 30–60°.
Grade III: severe >60°.

Management

The treatment goals for SCFE are to prevent or correct femoral head deformity that might lead to early symptoms, gait abnormalities, and late osteoarthritis. This is achieved by interventions to achieve the following objectives:

1. Stabilise the physis, inducing closure to prevent further slip.
2. Minimize the eventual deformity by operative reduction or corrective osteotomy if necessary.
3. Avoid complications especially avascular necrosis (AVN).

Surgical options

In-Situ Fixation

- The goal is to prevent further slip.
- Percutaneous in-situ fixation with a single, cannulated screw has consistently shown good results and is widely used as the mainstay of treatment for mild and moderate slips.
- The screw should be located in the centre of the proximal femoral epiphysis on both the anteroposterior and lateral views and should be perpendicular to the physis.

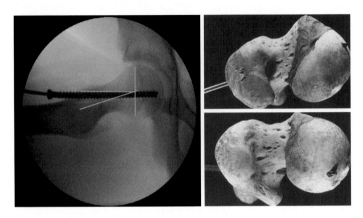

FIGURE 8.6 Intraoperative lateral radiograph and bone specimen highlighting the posterior slip of the femoral head and the necessary anterior neck entry point

- Because of the direction of the slip, it should be inserted from the anterior femoral neck in most cases in order to allow fixation perpendicular to the physis and to prevent hardware penetration through the posterior femoral neck (Fig. 8.6).
- As a result, severe slip pinning is more challenging. Screw entry point risks being intra-articular leading to impingement. There is an increased risk of posterior neck penetration and AVN and finally there is a greater chance of slip progression with less screw threads in the head providing stable fixation to prevent growing off.
- There are increasing rates of pin penetration and complications with an increasing number of screws.
- Articular screw penetration should not be missed as it may cause chrondrolysis and should be avoided.
- There is risk of subtrochanteric fracture due to low pin placement or following screw removal.
- In unstable slips a technique of urgent controlled gentle reduction, combined with capsulotomy and evacuation of haematoma followed by fixation with at least 2 wires or screws has been shown to be safe with a reduced rate of AVN compared to pinning in situ alone.

Realignment Osteotomy (Fish/Dunn/Modified Dunn)

- Osteotomies can be used by the experienced paediatric surgeon to perform a near anatomic reduction at the site of the slip with strategies to remove impediments to reduction and preserve blood flow. It is utilised in unstable and moderate to severe stable slips with open physes.
- Traditionally, this is performed via an anterolateral Watson-Jones (Dunn) approach with a trochanteric flip (Fig. 8.7) or an anterior modified Smith-Peterson (Fish) (Fig. 8.8) with a cuneiform subcapital osteotomy to reduce the neck onto the head with careful preservation of the posterior retinacular vessels. Results in the literature are encouraging although AVN rates up to 37% have been reported along with femoral neck shortening, leading to increased abductor force, increased joint pressures and very rarely instability. They are best performed in tertiary paediatric orthopaedic centres.
- Ganz and his colleagues described a modified Dunn procedure involving a trochanteric osteotomy with or without surgical hip dislocation to allow identification and protection

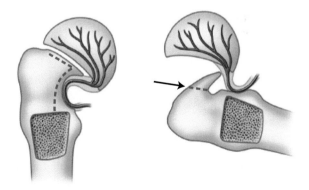

FIGURE 8.7 The Dunn procedure (1964). *Dotted line* represents the plane of separation of the epiphysis. The *arrow* indicates the posterior neck callus which requires resection in order to avoid tension on the retinacular vessels once the slip of the epiphysis is reduced

118   L. Jeyaseelan and K. James

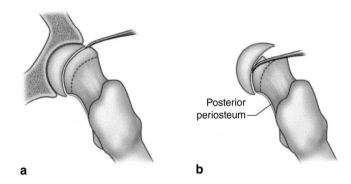

FIGURE 8.8 Fish cuneiform subcapital wedge resection. (a) A corrective osteotomy is performed first through the physis preserving posterior periosteum. (b) Secondly, a closing wedge resection of the anterior femoral neck allows correction of the posterior slip. The *dotted line* represents the outline of greater trochanter

of the deep branch of the medial femoral circumflex artery and retinacular vessels in order to preserve the blood supply to the epiphysis. The technique permits development of an extended retinacular flap and direct visualization and removal of callus on the posterior neck and other obstacles to anatomic reduction without tension on the blood supply. Controlled reduction of the femoral epiphysis can then be performed with fixation in a near anatomical position. This approach is technically demanding and evidence of its efficacy in reducing the avascular necrosis rate is limited to small cases series. There is however concern that the rate of AVN may be unacceptably high, even in specialist centres.

Other Proximal Femoral Osteotomies

The more distal the site of osteotomy, the lower the risk of AVN and chondrolysis.

Options include extracapsular/intertrochanteric osteotomies, which are the most commonly performed of the osteotomies. The three common components of the osteotomy are valgus, flexion, and internal rotation.

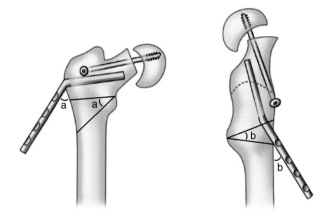

FIGURE 8.9 Extracapsular/intertrochanteric osteotomy. (**a**) Angle of wedge resection required to correct the neck shaft angle on the AP view, (**b**) angle of wedge resection required to correct the neck shaft angle on the lateral view

As the osteotomy is away from the CORA (centre of rotation and angulation) of the slip, the maximum degree of correction is limited to around 50–60° (Fig. 8.9).

Recommendation for intertrochanteric osteotomy can be made on the basis of clinical signs and symptoms or on a biomechanical basis in an attempt to normalise proximal femoral anatomy with the theoretical decrease in the long-term risk of OA.

Leg length discrepancy is a recognised side effect of the procedure.

Complications

Avascular Necrosis

The most significant complication is avascular necrosis of the femoral head. It may be a consequence of:

1. The natural history of some slips due immediate damage to the retinacular vessels or as a result of other factors: e.g.

delay in treatment secondary to increased intracapsular pressure from a haemarthrosis.

2. The treatment itself, in particular:

   A. The reduction manoeuvre (especially if posterior callus is present).
   B. The surgical approach; intracapsular osteotomies.
   C. Malposition screw/s in the femoral head.

The most important risk factor for AVN is stability of the physis:

- Unstable slips have reported AVN rates between 10 and 60%.
- Stable SCFEs have <1% AVN rate in slips that can be managed with single in situ screw fixation.

The unstable slip with severe displacement is at highest risk for AVN.

Avascular necrosis is associated with collapse of the femoral head and rapid progression of arthritis. There are currently no established treatments to prevent femoral head collapse with the majority of individuals affected requiring joint replacement as a young adult. The role of bisphosphonates is under investigations but its efficacy is undefined.

Chondrolysis

Progressive loss of articular cartilage is associated with penetration of the joint and spica cast immobilisation (although this is now rarely performed for SCFE). It occurs in up to 2% of cases and is characterised by pain, decreased hip range of motion, and radiographic joint space narrowing. It may be linked to femoral acetabular impingement.

Femoroacetabular Impingement (FAI)

Over half of SCFE patients undergoing arthroscopic evaluation have evidence of cartilage or labral damage. With increasing slip severity, the prominent anterior bump on the neck results in CAM type impingement, followed by mixed impingement, and in severe slips the bump is unable to enter into the acetabulum causing pincer type impingement (Fig. 8.10). In the future, the use of fixation devices that provides stability but allow continued growth thereby allowing remodelling of head-neck offset may well mitigate concerns over FAI. Currently, the role and indications of such devices are undefined.

Severe SCFE

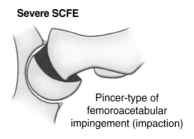

Pincer-type of femoroacetabular impingement (impaction)

Moderate SCFE

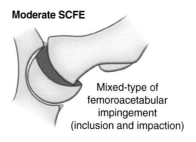

Mixed-type of femoroacetabular impingement (inclusion and impaction)

Mild SCFE

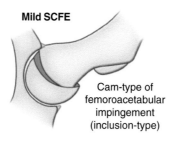

Cam-type of femoroacetabular impingement (inclusion-type)

FIGURE 8.10 Diagram showing the developing of FAI following a SCFE

Osteoarthritis/Natural History

Long term follow up studies have reported rates of hip pain in a third of patients with mild to moderate slips with 20% requiring joint replacement by 30 years.

Contralateral SCFE

The prevention of contralateral SUFE with prophylactic pinning has previously been controversial except in individuals with significant risk factors, such as endocrine abnormalities or considerable growth remaining to prevent leg length inequality. Recent studies have demonstrated that measurement of the posterior sloping angle to be useful tool in predicting future slip (Fig. 8.11). A Posterior sloping angle >14

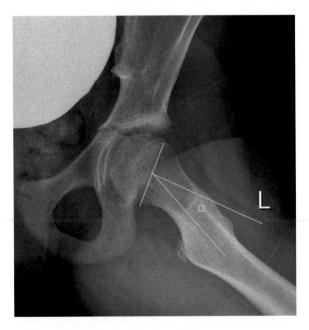

FIGURE 8.11 The posterior sloping angle is defined as the angle between the line along the plane of the physis and the line perpendicular to the femoral neck-diaphyseal axis on a frog leg lateral radiograph

has a number needed to treat of 1.79 to prevent a subsequent slip of the contralateral hip.

Synopsis

Slipped capital femoral epiphysis (SCFE) occurs following failure of the proximal femoral physis, resulting in displacement of the proximal femoral epiphysis relative to the femoral neck and shaft. Patients typically present between 12 and 14 years of age. Diagnosis can be made on AP and frog leg lateral radiographs. Treatment aims to prevent further slippage and reduce subsequent complications, including AVN, chondrolysis and osteoarthritis. This can be achieved through in-situ pinning, reduction and pinning or proximal femoral osteotomy, which may also be used for later deformity correction.

Key References

Ganz R, Parvizi J, Beck M, Leunig M, Nötzli H, Siebenrock KA. Femoroacetabular impingement: a cause for osteoarthritis of the hip. Clin Orthop Relat Res. 2003;417:112–20.

Hägglund G, Hansson LI, Sandström S. Slipped capital femoral epiphysis in southern Sweden. Long-term results after nailing/pinning. Clin Orthop Relat Res. 1987;217:190–200.

Leunig M, Slongo T, Ganz R. Subcapital realignment in slipped capital femoral epiphysis: surgical hip dislocation and trimming of the stable trochanter to protect the perfusion of the epiphysis. Instr Course Lect. 2008;57:499–507.

Ramachandran M, Ward K, Brown RR, Munns CF, Cowell CT, Little DG. Intravenous bisphosphonate therapy for traumatic osteonecrosis of the femoral head in adolescents. J Bone Joint Surg Am. 2007;89(8):1727–34.

Chapter 9
Congenital Coxa Vara

Stephen Key and Manoj Ramachandran

Definition

The neck shaft angle is the angle subtended by the axis of the femoral shaft with the axis of the femoral neck and is normally in the region of 150° in the infant, reducing to 125° in the adult. Coxa vara is a deformity of the proximal femur with a neck-shaft angle of less than 120°.

Coxa vara is associated with reduced femoral neck anteversion and defective ossification in the inferior femoral neck. It may be a true congenital abnormality (present from birth), developmental (autosomal dominant and progressive), or acquired. Controversy exists in the literature about the classification and nomenclature of this condition; the main focus of this chapter will be the primary forms of coxa vara, both congenital and developmental, with no other identified cause.

S. Key, MA, MBBChir, MRCS (Eng)
T&O SpR Royal London Rotation, London, UK

M. Ramachandran, BSc, MBBS, FRCS (T&O) (✉)
Paediatric and Young Adult Orthopaedic Unit, The Royal London and Barts and The London Children's Hospitals, Barts Health, London, UK
e-mail: manojorthopod@gmail.com

N.A. Aresti et al. (eds.), *Paediatric Orthopaedics in Clinical Practice*, In Clinical Practice,
DOI 10.1007/978-1-4471-6769-3_9,
© Springer-Verlag London 2016

Epidemiology

- Rare – 1/25,000 live births.
- Both sides are equally affected.
- Bilateral in 30–50%.
- Males and females equally affected.
- There is a familial predisposition – autosomal dominant inheritance of developmental coxa vara, in addition to heritability of associated skeletal dysplasias.

Aetiology

The main controversy in the literature concerns the aetiological classification of this condition. Broadly, the primary forms, with no other cause, are considered to be either congenital or developmental, while those with an obvious underlying cause are acquired. Different authors use various definitions for these terms but we present one commonly used system:

- *Congenital* – significant varus deformity present at birth, assumed to be due to limb bud abnormality in the developing embryo.

  - Associations:

    - Proximal femoral focal deficiency.
    - Congenital short femur.
    - Congenital bowed femur.

Confusion exists around the classification of coxa vara in association with inherited skeletal dysplasias. Some authors consider these to be primary congenital forms of the disease, while others consider them to be acquired. The major inherited dysplasias with which coxa vara is associated are (see Chap. 14):

- Multiple epiphyseal dysplasia.
- Spondyloepiphyseal dysplasia congenita.
- Chondrodysplasia punctata.
- Metaphyseal chondrodysplasia.
- Achondroplasia.
- Cleidocranial dysostosis.

- *Developmental* – Autosomal dominant disorder. The proximal femur is normal at birth but progressive varus deformity develops in early childhood.
- *Acquired* – Deformity develops secondary to other bone pathology, which typically causes bone softening or fracture.

  – Biochemical:

    - Rickets.
    - Renal osteodystrophy.

  – Sequelae of avascular necrosis:

    - Legg-Calve-Perthes' disease.
    - Traumatic – femoral neck fracture or traumatic dislocation of hip.
    - Post-reduction for developmental dysplasia of the hip.
    - Slipped capital femoral epiphysis.

  – Infection:

    - TB or pyogenic.

  – Skeletal dysplasias:

    - Fibrous dysplasia.
    - Osteogenesis imperfecta.
    - Osteopetrosis.

Pathogenesis

The underlying pathogenesis of primary coxa vara is unknown, and likely to be multifactorial. Possible theories include:

1. Metabolic abnormality – deficiency in proximal femur ossification.
2. Excessive intrauterine pressure – causes depression in femoral neck.
3. Non-specific mechanical abnormality – occurs during development.

4. Vascular insult – arrest in neck development.
5. Localized dysplasia – faulty maturation of cartilage & bone in femoral neck.

Histological abnormalities have been identified in the medial physis and adjacent metaphyseal bone. Characteristically, the physis is widened and there is disordered progress of the cartilage columns. The adjacent metaphyseal bone is porotic and contains nests of cartilage.

It is thought that the primary deformity is caused by defective ossification in the inferior femoral neck. Shearing stresses produced during weight bearing through the vertically oriented physis, then fatigue the abnormal bone and cartilage leading to progression of the deformity. Not only does the orientation of the physis change, but consistent with the Heuter-Volkmann law, increased compressive forces at the medial physis inhibit medial growth of the neck, while lateral growth is stimulated by increased tensile forces.

Symptoms and Signs

Primary coxa vara usually presents after a child begins to walk, most between the ages of 2–6 years, with a painless limp and leg length discrepancy when unilateral, or a waddling gait if bilateral. This is due to abductor insufficiency secondary to mechanical disadvantage caused by the deformity. There may be a positive Trendelenburg sign. Examination of torsional profile will demonstrate reduced femoral anteversion, or possible retroversion. Range of movement is reduced particularly in abduction and internal rotation.

Evidence of a generalised skeletal dysplasia should be sought, especially in the presence of bilateral coxa vara, short stature, or a positive family history.

Investigations

Plain AP radiographs are used to make the diagnosis and assess the severity of the deformity (Fig. 9.1). The neck-shaft angle lies between the axes of the femoral neck and femoral shaft and is, by definition, less than 120°. The physis is vertically oriented and can be quantified by the head-shaft angle between the shaft axis and the perpendicular to

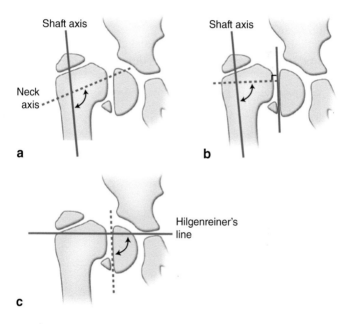

FIGURE 9.1 A diagram demonstrating the parameters for measuring the extent of the deformity in the proximal femur: (**a**) The neck shaft angle, i.e. the angle between the shaft and neck. (**b**) The head shaft angle, i.e. the angle between the perpendicular to the line drawn along the base of the upper femoral epiphysis and the femoral shaft. (**c**) Hilgenreiner's angle, i.e. the angle between Hilgenreiner's line and the line drawn along the base of the upper femoral ephiphysis

the base of the capital femoral epiphysis. The Hilgenreiner-epiphyseal angle lies between Hilgenreiner's line and a line parallel to the capital femoral physis; this angle is used to guide treatment and should normally be less than 25°.

In addition to the varus deformity, the neck is short (coxa breva) and the physis widened. There is reduced proximal femoral anteversion or retroversion, and the acetabulum may be dysplastic. Fairbank's triangle is a sclerotic ossification defect in the inferomedial metaphysis, surrounded by a radiolucent inverted "Y" of dystrophic bone; when present this is pathognomonic for developmental coxa vara (Fig. 9.2).

Further investigations specific to skeletal dysplasias and acquired causes are performed as required.

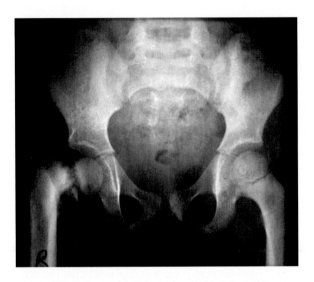

FIGURE 9.2 AP radiograph of a patient with idiopathic coxa vara affecting the right hip. Note the difference in aforementioned parameters between the two hips and the presence of Fairbank's triangle

Prognosis

For primary coxa vara, progression is dependent on the Hilgenreiner-epiphyseal angle:

- <45° defect will usually heal spontaneously and will not progress.
- 45–60° – may progress but needs close observation.
- >60° will progress.

In acquired forms there should be minimal risk of progression provided the underlying cause is corrected.

Treatment

This is also based on Hilgenreiner-epiphyseal angle:

- <45° – no treatment required – should resolve spontaneously.
- 45–60° – observe – consider osteotomy if severe gait abnormality or progressive.
- >60° – valgus osteotomy.

A valgus osteotomy can be performed at the sub- or intertrochanteric level, aiming for an overcorrection to a neckshaft angle of at least 150°, and an epiphyseal angle of less than 30–40°. Rotation should also be corrected to 10–20° anteversion; this requires at least 20° of external rotation pre-operatively.

Many different osteotomies and methods of fixation have been described. The goal of surgery, however, is always to correct the varus and torsional deformities, while correcting leg length discrepancy and repositioning the physis from a vertical to a more horizontal position, to convert loading from shear to compressive stress (Fig. 9.3). This encourages healing of the femoral neck ossification defect and ultimately, correct abductor tension improves gait. The osteotomy is held

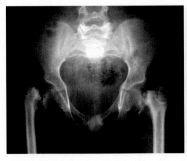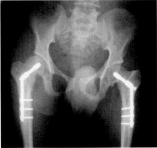

FIGURE 9.3 Example of correction of coxa vara and fixation using locked sliding hip screws and plates

in place by internal fixation followed by 6 weeks in a hip spica post-operatively in the young child. Healing of the metaphyseal defect can be expected within 3–6 months if sufficient valgus is achieved.

Other procedures that may be required:

- Adductor tenotomy may be required to increase abduction, required for valgus osteotomy.
- Trochanteric advancement in the case of trochanteric overgrowth, to correct abductor tension.
- Greater trochanteric apophyseodesis to prevent trochanteric overgrowth associated with premature physeal closure. This has previously been used as sole treatment but was found unreliable when used alone.
- Correction of leg length discrepancy when severe.

Complications

- Loss of correction – related to undercorrection and may require repeat osteotomy. Recurrence of the deformity is estimated between 30 and 70%.
- Premature capital physeal closure – seen in up to 90% of operated hips and associated with trochanteric overgrowth (may require apophyseodesis or trochanteric advancement) and acetabular dysplasia.

Summary

Coxa vara is a rare deformity of the proximal femur characterised by reduced neck-shaft angle, associated with reduced femoral anteversion, causing abductor insufficiency. It may be congenital, developmental or acquired. The primary forms usually present before 6 years of age. Diagnosis is made by plain AP radiographs of the pelvis and treatment is determined by measurement of the Hilgenreiner-epiphyseal angle, with valgus osteotomy indicated where this is greater than 60°, or 45–60° and progressive with marked gait abnormality.

Historical Note

The first clinical description of congenital coxa vara was produced by Fiorani in 1881. The term coxa vara was first used by Hofmeister in 1884 after showing radiographic evidence of reduced neck-shaft angle. Progression of the deformity observed in childhood was noted by Fairbank in 1928, while Duncan in 1938 was the first to distinguish developmental coxa vara, absent at birth but progressive during childhood, from true congenital coxa vara, supported by the work of Amstutz in 1970.

Key References

Amstutz HC. Developmental (infantile) coxa vara — a distinct entity. Report of two patients with previously normal roentgenograms. Clin Orthop. 1970;72:242–7.

Bos CF, Sakkers RJ, Bloem JL, et al. Histological, biochemical, and MRI studies of the growth plate in congenital coxa vara. J Pediatr Orthop. 1989;9(6):660–5.

Pauwels F. Biomechanics of the normal and diseased hip. New York: Springer; 1979.

Weinstein JN, Kuo KN, Millar EA. Congenital coxa vara. A retrospective review. J Pediatr Orthop. 1984;4(1):70–7.

Chapter 10
Paediatric Knee

Jagwant Singh, Sam Heaton, and Kyle James

Synopsis

This chapter covers the paediatric conditions relating to the knee and proximal tibia. Whereas normal variants of alignment of the knee are covered in another chapter, here we will consider pathological causes.

Blount's disease involves the posteromedial portion of the tibial growth plate. Depending on the age of onset, it is classified as early (2–5 years) and late (over 10 years). Treatment depends on the age and deformity and ranges from bracing in children less than 3 years old to surgical intervention in older patients with progressive deformity. This chapter also gives an overview of patellar instability and Osteochondritis Dissecans (OCD).

J. Singh, MBBS, MRCS
T&O SpR Royal London Rotation, London, UK

S. Heaton, FRCS (Tr&Orth)
T&O SpR Royal London Rotation, London, UK

K. James, FRCS (Tr&Orth) (✉)
Paediatric and Young Adult Orthopaedic Unit,
The Royal London and Barts and The London Children's
Hospitals, Barts Health, London, UK
e-mail: kyledimitrijames@gmail.com

N.A. Aresti et al. (eds.), *Paediatric Orthopaedics
in Clinical Practice*, In Clinical Practice,
DOI 10.1007/978-1-4471-6769-3_10,
© Springer-Verlag London 2016

Patellar instability in skeletally immature patients can be grouped into acute dislocations and recurrent patellofemoral instability. Acute patellar dislocations are treated primarily by immobilisation; acute surgery is only indicated in cases of associated osteochondral fracture. Multiple surgical options have been described for chronic instability.

OCD is a subchondral bone pathology that affects the cartilage eventually. It is important to differentiate between stable and unstable lesions with the latter usually requiring some form of surgical intervention. Surgery is either reparative (fixation or drilling) or restorative (microfracture, ACI, OATS, excision or allograft).

Malalignment Conditions

Causes of genu valgum (knock-knees) may be categorized as physiological or pathological, and sub-categorized as unilateral or bilateral:

- Physiological – Normal from 2 years onwards (bilateral) – see Chapter 1 (Normal variants and self-limiting conditions).
- Pathological:

  - Idiopathic (unilateral or bilateral).
  - Post-traumatic (unilateral).
  - Metabolic e.g. rickets, renal osteodystrophy (bilateral).
  - Neuromuscular (unilateral or bilateral).
  - Post-infection (unilateral).
  - Congenital (e.g. pseudoachondroplasia).
  - Skeletal dysplasias e.g. multiple epiphyseal dysplasia (bilateral).
  - Benign tumours e.g. Ollier's disease, osteochondromas, fibrocartilaginous dysplasia (unilateral).

Causes of genu varum (bow-legs) may be similarly categorized:

- Persistent physiological varus – Becomes more apparent when 2 years old.

– Pathological:

- Idiopathic (unilateral or bilateral).
- Blount's disease.
- Fibrocartilaginous dysplasia.
- Metabolic e.g. hypophosphatemic/vitamin D deficiency rickets, renal osteodystrophy (bilateral).
- Post-traumatic (unilateral).
- Post-infection (unilateral).
- Benign tumours e.g. osteochondromas (unilateral).
- Metaphyseal chondrodysplasia.
- Spondyloepiphyseal or metaphyseal-epiphyseal dysplasias.

In severe adolescent Blount's, hypoplasia of the distal femoral medial condyle results in distal femoral varus. The significance of femoral varus should be determined preoperatively in late onset Blount's disease to avoid compensatory deformity.

Blount's Disease

Blount's disease (tibia vara) is a developmental disorder of unknown cause that primarily affects the medial portion of the proximal tibial growth plate and if left untreated can lead to permanent (normally varus) deformity and osteoarthritis.

Historical Notes

Erlacher in 1922 first identified Tibia Vara but it was W.P. Blount, a physician from Milwaukee, Wisconsin who fully described this condition in 1937 as "osteochondrosis deformans tibia".

Pathology

The pathophysiology is based on the Heuter-Volkmann principle of growth inhibition caused by excessive compressive forces and is often bilateral. Based on age at clinical onset and distinct features, Blount's disease has been classified into:

- Early or infantile.
- Late or adolescent.

Blount's is caused by a multifactorial, mechanical overload in genetically susceptible individuals. This leads to excessive medial pressure producing osteochondrosis of the medial proximal tibial physis and epiphysis.

Spontaneous growth suppression of the posteromedial proximal tibial physis results in varus, flexion and internal rotation deformity. This leads to medial and posterior sloping of the proximal tibial epiphysis and increased deformity of the proximal tibia and distal femur eventually causing knee laxity and instability. The varus deformity progresses as long as ossification is defective and growth continues laterally.

There is disruption of normal columnar architecture of the physis, and replacement of physeal cartilage by fibrous tissue. The severe forms of Blount's disease is characterised by physeal arrest and bar formation between the epiphysis and metaphysis.

Early walking age, obesity and Vitamin D deficiency have been shown to be the predisposing factors. Hispanic and black children have a greater predilection.

Early Blount's Disease

Early Blount's typically affect children aged 2–5. It tends to affect obese black children who are early walkers.

Clinical Features

Children present with the following features:

- Varus deformity of the proximal tibia.
- Increased internal tibial torsion.
- Beaking or prominence of their proximal medial tibial epiphysis.
- Leg length inequality (in unilateral cases).
- Around 50% of patients present with bilateral deformity that is not necessarily symmetrical.

In addition to varus deformity, the extent of physeal and epiphyseal involvement varies. Langenskiold described the radiographic classification system as shown in Fig. 10.1. However it cannot be relied on for prognosis. Of note, changes typical of tibia vara do not appear before the age of 1 year.

The metaphyseal-diaphyseal angle (MDA) or Drennan's angle assessed on an AP radiograph can be used to differentiate between physiological varus and infantile Blount's disease (Figs. 10.2 and 10.3).

- Angles <11° suggests physiological genu varum.
- Angles of >16° suggests Blount's disease.
- Those in between with medial beaking are more likely to progress to true infantile Blount's disease and should be closely monitored.

Management

A simple algorithm for treatment is as follows:

- Patients ≤3 years. who are Langenskiold's stage I/II can be initially treated conservatively in a long leg anti-varus brace during the day.
- Those ≥4 years, with progressive radiographic deformity or Langenskiold's stage III–IV are likely to require surgery.

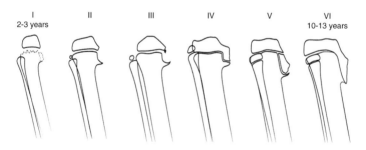

FIGURE 10.1 Langenskiold's radiographic classification of infantile Blount disease. Progressive stages from mild medial epiphyseal-metaphyseal beaking (*stage I*) to complete medial proximal tibial physeal arrest (*stage VI*) (Reproduced with permission from *Tachdjian's pediatric orthopaedics* 4th Edition, 2nd volume)

Metaphyseal diaphyseal angle

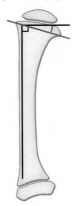

FIGURE 10.2 The tibial metaphyseal-diaphyseal angle (MDA), created by the intersection of a line connecting the most prominent medial portion of the proximal tibial metaphysis (the "beak") and the most prominent lateral point of the metaphysis with a line drawn perpendicular to the long axis of the tibial diaphysis

Surgical options include the following:

- High tibial osteotomy – The goal is correct the varus, flexion, and internal rotational deformities of the tibia. By reducing the weight bearing across the medial joint, growth and subsequent correction of the deformity ensues. The younger the patient, the greater the risk of recurrence, hence overcorrection is common. Correction can be achieved with acute or staged osteotomies and with immediate internal fixation or treatment with a frame. An oblique osteotomy can be used to correct both the varus and internal rotation components of the deformity (Fig. 10.4).
- In severe cases, a medial hemiplateau elevation osteotomy may be required.
- The use of guided growth plates can be used to perform a hemiephysiodesis/growth modulation. Satisfactory results have been observed with this technique, although metalwork failure remains an issue.

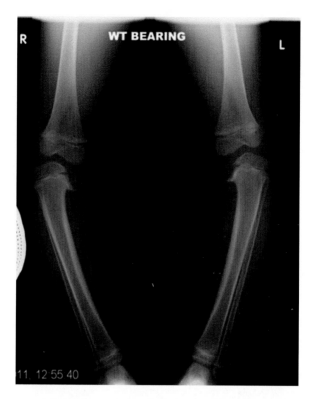

FIGURE 10.3 Long leg radiograph showing bilateral Blount's disease

Complications

Possible complications from surgery include the following:

- Compartment syndrome.
- Nerve injury (common peroneal nerve).
- Infection.
- Malunion/nonunion.
- Recurrence.
- Physeal arrest.

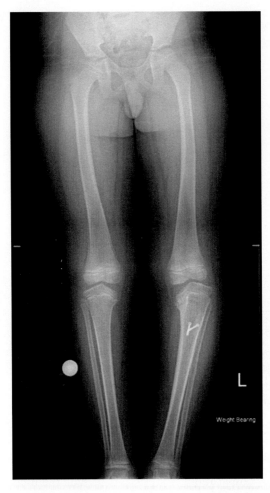

FIGURE 10.4 Radiographs show reoccurrence after high tibial oste-otomy

Late Blount's Disease

The less common and less severe adolescent form of Blount's affects children over the age of 10 and is typically associated with obesity. Excess weight is thought to cause overloading of the medial joint on an already mildly varus knee (Fig. 10.5).

Features associated with the adolescent form include:

- A greater chance of unilateral cases, possibly increasing limb length discrepancy.
- Distal femoral physeal growth disturbances, exacerbating the varus deformity.

Typical radiographic features include:

- Associated femoral deformity (usually valgus).
- Widening of the **medial** tibial physis.
- Widening of the **lateral** femoral physis.
- Narrowing of the tibial epiphysis.
- Beaking is not as common as the infantile type.
- As with infantile Blount's, the MDA is greater than 16°.

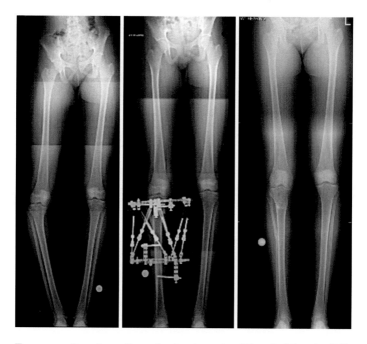

FIGURE 10.5 Long leg radiographs showing an late Blount's deformity (*left*), corrected using a frame (*middle*) and post-treatment alignment (*right*)

Management

In untreated cases, deformity worsens and early osteoarthritis sets in due to altered joint kinematics. Reversal of the driving force (obesity) should be addressed but as there is less potential for remodeling due to age, non-operative treatment is of limited value and poor outcomes are typically seen in all but mild cases.

As with infantile Blount's, surgery typically involves correction via a proximal tibial osteotomy. Once again, this can be acute or gradual and fixed acutely or using a frame. Overcorrection is not required at this advanced age, as ensuing growth tends to be along the mechanical axis. In some patients with enough remaining growth potential, hemiepiphysiodesis remains an option. Treatment of femoral deformity by similar methods may also be considered.

Recurrence of deformity following a high tibial osteotomy implies severe and possibly irreversible medial proximal tibial physeal growth disturbances. In these cases, future treatment has to be individualized taking into account the age, deformity, joint distortion and leg length inequality.

Focal Fibrocartilaginous Dysplasia (FFCD)

FFCD is a rare and benign condition affecting the proximal tibia of toddlers and infants (Fig. 10.6). It has the same prevalence in both sexes. The clinical features of tibial FFCD include:

    Painless unilateral tibia vara.
- Medial tibial torsion.
- Leg length discrepancy.
- Limping or normal walking.

It is a result of failure of differentiation of the mesenchymal anlage in the area of the pes anserinus. Persistence of a fibrocartilage focus hampers growth on the medial aspect of proximal tibia. Given the physis is normal, the deformity typically corrects. In the rare cases where it doesn't, correction may be achieved by curettage of the lesion.

Congenital Dislocation of the Knee (CDK)

Congenital dislocation of the knee or "back knee" comprises of a spectrum of deformities ranging from subluxation to complete dislocation. The incidence is estimated at 1 per 100,00 live births.

It often occurs in association with:

– Arthrogryposis multiplex congenital (AMC).
– Larsen's syndrome.
– Musculoskeletal anomalies such as DDH and clubfoot.

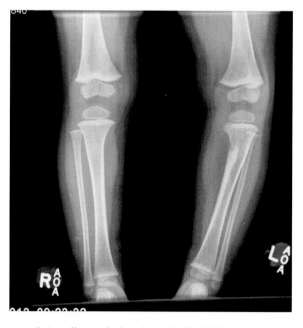

FIGURE 10.6 A radiograph showing left sided tibia vara as a result of Focal Fibrocartilaginous Dysplasia

The features of CDK include:

– A typical position of recurvatum of the knee.
– Shortening of the quadriceps tendon.
– Tight anterior capsule.
– Hypoplasia of the suprapatellar bursa.
– Valgus deformity is noted in half of CDK cases.

Laurence classified congenital knee dislocations into three 3 grades: grade I (severe genu recurvatum), grade II (subluxation), or grade III (complete dislocation).

Treatment normally involves manipulation via manual traction until the tibia is felt to engage with the femoral condyles, followed by flexion of the knee. Serial casting in progressive flexion should then be performed. If commenced at an early stage (before 3 months), conservative treatment is likely to succeed. In older children with a moderate to severe subluxation or dislocation, surgery is indicated and will give a satisfactory result if performed within 2 years, although the optimal time is at 6 months. Early closed reduction (within 24 h.) has shown good to excellent results.

Patellar Instability

Patella instability is a multi-factorial process that affects females greater than males (3:1 ratio). Recurrent dislocation/ ensuing instability is present in 15–20% of cases following a first episode of patellar dislocation. Younger children (<14 years) are more likely to develop recurrent dislocations than older children.

Patella stability relies on:

– Bone structure, i.e. the shape of the patella and trochlear. Bone structure is most important in deep knee flexion.
– Muscle action provides dynamic stability, directly and predominantly through vastus medialis, but also via hip muscles, particularly gluteus maximus, adductors and TFL.
– Ligaments, namely the medial patellofemoral ligament (MPFL), control the first 20° of flexion.

Given the complex anatomy that provides patella stability, it is unsurprising that instability is multi-factorial. Dejour described four main factors that contribute to instability, although this may be more applicable to the adult knee. These are:

– Trochlea dysplasia.
– Quadriceps dysplasia.
– Patella alta.
– Tibial tuberosity-trochlear groove of >20 mm (Fig. 10.7).

Other risk factors that may contribute to dislocation include:

– Excessive external femoral and tibial rotation.
– Genu recurvatum.
– Genu valgum.
– Generalized ligament laxity.
– Patella maldevelopment (patella alta).
– Miserable malalignment syndrome – the combination of femoral anteversion, genu valgum and external tibial torsion, which leads to patellofemoral malalignment with an increased Q angle (Fig. 10.8).

Clinical Assessment

Patients may present with anterior knee pain alone, or pain associated with subluxation/dislocation of their patella. Acute presentations may be associated with an effusion/haemarthrosis and tenderness over the MPFL. Further clinical examination may reveal patellar apprehension, an increase in passive patellar translation and abnormal patellar tracking (J-sign). Beighton's score is useful in assessing ligament laxity.

Investigations

Radiographs help to rule out a loose body or fracture and may help identify factors contributing to recurrent dislocation of the patella.

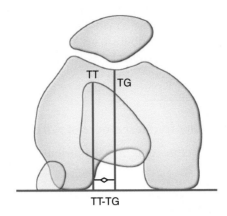

FIGURE 10.7 The TTTG distance, measured on an axial CT, is the distance between two perpendicular lines – one from the posterior cortex to the tibial tubercle (*TT*) and the other across the trochlear groove (*TG*). A TT TG distance of >20 mm is considered abnormal

Management

Acute patellar dislocations commonly spontaneously reduce. If they present still dislocated, manipulation with gentle knee flexion to ensure the patella engages in the trochlea is advised. Evacuation of the haemarthrosis +/− infiltration of the knee with local anaesthetic may relieve symptoms dramatically.

Isolated dislocations, once reduced, are treated with initial immobilisation (for pain alone) followed by early physical therapy focusing on quadriceps, core and hip strengthening. Surgery is only indicated in cases with an associated osteo-chondral fracture.

Indications for surgery include:

- Associated osteochondral fracture.
- Severe instability with dislocation in every flexion arc.

Several options exist in the surgical management. They include:

• Lateral retinaculum release with medial retinaculum imbrication.

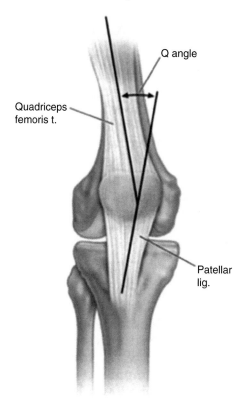

FIGURE 10.8 The Q angle is the angle formed by a line drawn from the anterior superior iliac spine to the centre of the patella and a second line drawn from the centre of the patella to tibial tubercle. A large Q angle is associated with a tendency toward lateral subluxation of the patella. The normal Q-angle is 15° in females and 10° in males (Reproduced with permission from *Tachdjian's pediatric orthopaedics* 4th Edition, 2nd volume)

- MPFL reconstruction using techniques that avoid tunnel or screw fixation around the distal femoral physis.
- Roux-Goldthwait procedure, which involves transposition of the lateral half of the patella tendon under the medial half and sutured to the periosteum medially.

In patients with increased Q-angles, distal realignment procedures that may impact on open physes, such as tibial tuberosity transfers, are contraindicated as they may cause growth disturtbances and deformity.

Osteochondritis Dissecans (OCD)

Definition

OCD is a pathological condition affecting subchondral bone with secondary damage to the overlying articular cartilage. If left untreated, a loss of continuity can lead to degenerative arthritis due to joint incongruity and abnormal wear patterns.

Epidemiology

Two forms of OCD exist: juvenile or adult. Juvenile OCD occurs in children and adolescents with open growth plates, usually between 10 and 15 years. The adult form presents after skeletal maturity and has a much poorer prognosis.

Aetiology

Avascular necrosis of the bone is the characteristic pathologic finding. The hyaline cartilage appears normal at first but it undergoes degenerative changes, including softening, fibrillation, and fissuring when subchondral bony support is lost.

Multiple theories exist with no conclusive evidence for any one cause. Hypotheses include:

- Repetitive trauma.
- Genetic factors.
- Ischaemia.
- Failure to fuse of a normal accessory ossification centre.
- Inflammation.

Presentation

Affected children may or may not give a history of trauma. The OCD may be incidental when another injury is investigated or be the primary cause of symptoms. Possible symptoms may include:

– Generalized knee pain.
– An effusion (less than 20%).
– Mechanical symptoms e.g. catching, locking and giving way.

Physical examination may show an antalgic gait with point tenderness over the affected area. A positive Wilson's sign is when internal tibia rotation during extension from 90° to 30° elicits pain, which is relieved by external rotation. The Wilson test is of poor diagnostic value with only 16% positive tests in knees with proven OCDs. Unstable lesions may give crepitus while chronic lesions may lead to quadriceps atrophy.

Investigations

Imaging is essential for a diagnosis. Plain radiographs should include an AP standing film and 45° flexion PA/tunnel views (which show the posterior condyles), lateral and patella skyline views (Fig. 10.9). Bilateral radiographs should be requested due to common bilateral knee involvement.

Berndt and Hearty classified the radiograph findings, initially based on talar OCD lesions, into four types:

• Stage I – Small area of subchondral bone compression.
• Stage II – Partially detached fragment.
• Stage III – Completely detached fragment, remains in crater.
• Stage IV – Complete detachment, loose body (Fig. 10.10).

Once the OCD has been diagnosed using plain radiographs, or is suspected, then an MRI is routinely used in order to define the following features (Fig. 10.11):

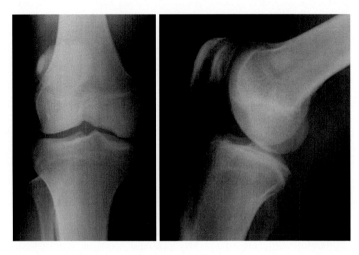

FIGURE 10.9 Anterior posterior and lateral radiographs of the knee in a skeletally mature patient showing the classical area for OCD on the lateral aspect of the medial femoral condyle

- Geometry (size, depth, location).
- Stability – evidence of linear high-intensity signals on T2 sequences between the lesion and parent bone – particularly useful in guiding treatment.
- Presence of loose bodies and subchondral bone evaluation.
- State of the articular cartilage (fissuring, thickness, water content, etc.).

Treatment

Treatment depends both on skeletal maturity (physeal closure) and lesion stability.

Non operative

Non-operative management with restrictive weight bearing and bracing should be the first-line treatment for

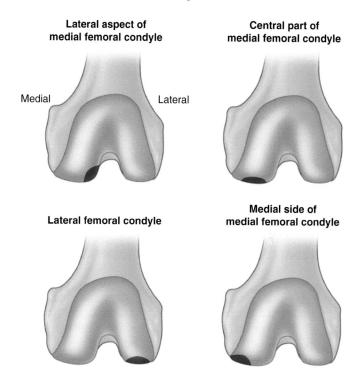

FIGURE 10.10 OCD most commonly involves the distal femur. Specific sites affected, include the lateral aspect of medial femoral condyle (51%) (see Fig. 10.9), the central part of medial femoral condyle (19%), the lateral femoral condyle (17%), the medial side of medial femoral condyle (7%) and the patella (7%)

stable OCD lesions in children. This modality is hugely varied with no strong evidence for any particular protocol. Options include the use of cylinder casts to a more liberal hiatus from sports and high impact activities. Approximately 50% heal by 10–18 months. Non-operative treatment should be adhered to for at least 3–6 months, after which persistent symptoms may warrant surgical intervention.

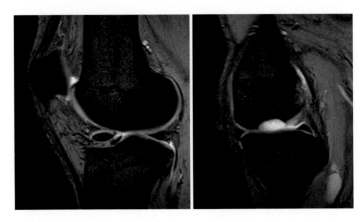

FIGURE 10.11 Sagittal MRI scan showing loose body and large defect, Diplaola grade IV. Note that this is the same patient as in Fig. 10.9

A European Paediatric Orthopaedic Society multicenter study of 509 knees demonstrated improved prognosis in young patients without dissection or an effusion, and with a lesion less than 2 cm² in a classical location (lateral aspect of the medial femoral condyle) when treated non-operatively. However in cases of chondral separation, surgery was better.

Operative

As eluded to above, surgery is indicated for:

– Unstable OCD lesions.
– Stable lesions that have failed a trial of non-operative treatment.

There are many surgical options but they can be broadly broken down in to reparative or restorative.

Reparative

The purpose here is to restore the subchondral interface thereby preserving the articular cartilage. The options here are:

- **Drilling.** The aim is to drill into subchondral bone, thereby creating vascular channels to devitalized areas and subsequent neovascularization. This brings in stem cells and inflammatory mediators, which encourage ossification.
- **Internal fixation.** High grade and unstable lesions presenting with loose bodies or cartilage flaps are more amenable to fixation than drilling.

Restorative

If the lesion is not amenable to fixation because of fragmentation, poor quality, incongruence or failure of healing after previous treatment then the options include

- **Fragment excision.** May alleviate symptoms initially but leads to degenerative findings on radiographs at 11 years postoperatively in approximately 79%.
- **Microfracture.**
- **Autologous chondrocyte implantation (ACI).** This involves a two stage operation with arthroscopic cartilage harvesting of non-articulating cartilage followed by open transplant of chondrocytes with various fixation methods around 6 weeks later.
- **Osteoarticular transfer system (OATS).** Useful when subchondral bone integrity is significantly compromised. When compared to microfracture, OATS has been found to have similar initial clinical improvements but better long-term results.

- **Osteochondral allograft.** Fresh osteochondral allograft is a salvage procedure suitable for large and deep OCDs and is rarely used as a first line treatment.

Key References

Blount WP. Tibia vara, osteochondrosis deformans tibiae. Curr Pract Orthop Surg. 1965;3:141–56.

Langenskiold A. Tibia vara. A critical review. Clin Orthop Relat Res. 1989;(246):195–207.

Vavken P, Wimmer MD, Camathias C, Quidde J, Valderrabano V, Pagenstert G. Treating patella instability in skeletally immature patients. Arthroscopy. 2013;29(8):1410–22.

Chambers HG, Shea KG, Carey JL. AAOS Clinical Practice Guideline: diagnosis and treatment of osteochondritis dissecans. J Am Acad Orthop Surg. 2011;19:307–9.

Chapter 11
Foot and Ankle

Alexander Charalambous and Matthew Barry

Introduction

Foot and ankle problems in children are a common cause of parental anxiety. It is important to distinguish a true deformity from a normal variant and to begin appropriate treatment promptly. The problem may be isolated or exist as part of an underlying condition. It is therefore important to consider this when performing your initial assessment. This chapter outlines common conditions and also some common normal variants.

A. Charalambous, MBChB, BSc (Hons), MRCS
T&O SpR Royal London Rotation,London, UK

M. Barry, MS, FRCS (Orth) (✉)
Paediatric and Young Adult Orthopaedic Unit,
The Royal London and The London Children's Hospitals,
Barts Health NHS Trust, London, UK
e-mail: matthew.barry@bartshealth.nhs.uk

N.A. Aresti et al. (eds.), *Paediatric Orthopaedics
in Clinical Practice*, In Clinical Practice,
DOI 10.1007/978-1-4471-6769-3_11,
© Springer-Verlag London 2016

Metatarsus Adductus

Epidemiology

Metatarsus adductus varies in its severity. It is present in up to 1 per 1000 births. It has equal incidence in both the sexes and is bilateral in up to half of cases. The aetiology is not clear but is linked to first pregnancy, twin pregnancy and oligohydramnios, suggesting packaging to be a cause.

Symptoms and Signs

The condition is rarely noted at birth, but during the first few months of life. The deformity is at the level of the tarsometatarsal joints and it is related to the intra-uterine position of the fetus. There is a strong association with developmental dysplasia of the hip (DDH) and therefore routine screening should be considered in these patients. Clinically, parents will note in-toeing. Differential diagnoses include congenital talipes equinovarus (CTEV), tibial torsion and femoral neck anteversion. Distinguish by careful examination (Fig. 11.1):

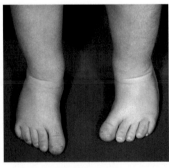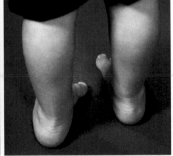

FIGURE 11.1 Metatarsus adductus. Note the adducted hallux and forefoot and the slightly valgus hindfoot (Reproduced from Benson et al. *Children's Orthopaedics and Fractures*, 2009, Springer)

- The forefoot is adducted and often supinated.
- Look at the lateral border of the foot for medial deviation.
- Check for deep medial skin creases in severe deformity.
- Check if the deformity is correctable.
- Check the hindfoot, which will be in neutral or valgus, compared to the varus position in CTEV.
- Examine all joints of the lower limb.
- Look for DDH.

A rare severe form of metatarsus adductus is seen in the 'serpentine (Z) foot' or 'severe skew foot' (Fig. 11.2). This is characterised by a rigid adduction deformity, with lateral subluxation of the navicular and hindfoot valgus.

Treatment

The majority of cases will resolve spontaneously. Any initial intervention should be in the form of stretches, moving to manipulation and serial casting if required. Length of treatment is variable but is often at least 10 weeks (Table 11.1). The goal is to achieve a straight lateral border of the foot.

Complication rates for surgical intervention are high and surgery is reserved for recurrent cases with severe deformity or late presentation. The fixed deformity seen in a Z foot often requires surgical intervention.

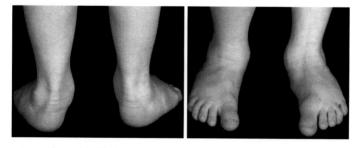

FIGURE 11.2 Serpentine deformity or Z-Foot (Reproduced from Benson et al. *Children's Orthopaedics and Fractures*, 2009, Springer)

TABLE 11.1 Initial treatment options in metatarsus adductus

Deformity correctable actively	No intervention required
Deformity correctable passively	Stretching exercises by parents
Rigid deformity or deep medial skin crease	Manipulation and serial casting

Surgical Intervention

- Soft tissue release: abductor hallucis longus recession or release with or without tibialis posterior lengthening. Joint capsulotomies are more invasive.
- Osteotomy: metatarsal open or closing wedge osteotomies can alter column length to correct fixed deformity where conservative therapy is not appropriate or has failed.

Metatarsus adductus

- Most cases resolve spontaneously.
- Use the hindfoot to distinguish from CTEV, the key differential not to be missed.
- Screen for DDH.

Talipes Calcaneovalgus

This deformity is more common in females and in first-born children (Fig. 11.3). It is often bilateral. Some cases are related to neurological conditions.

Symptoms and Signs

This condition presents shortly after birth. In contrast to CTEV, the hindfoot lies in a valgus position, with the foot dorsiflexed.

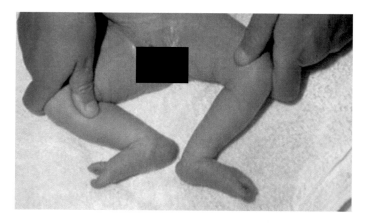

FIGURE 11.3 Calcaneovalgus feet in an infant (Reproduced from Benson et al. *Children's Orthopaedics and Fractures*, 2009, Springer)

- Look for skin creases anterior to the ankle.
- Dorsiflexion can be marked, with the dorsal surface of the foot lying in contact with the tibia.
- The deformity should be correctable passively.

Neurological examination is recommended as muscle imbalances caused by L5 spina bifida can cause this deformity. The condition is associated with DDH. Therefore, routine screening is recommended especially in unilateral cases. Other differential diagnoses include congenital postermedial tibial bowing and congenital vertical talus. Check if the deformity is fixed as expected in vertical talus.

Treatment

This deformity usually corrects spontaneously during the neonatal period. Severe deformity may require stretching exercises or serial casting.

Posteromedial Bowing of the Tibia

Posteromedial bowing of the tibia is a congenital disorder, which as its name suggests, leads to bowing of the tibia with the apex of the bow being posterior and medial. It normally affects the middle to distal portion of the tibia. The disorder is initially accompanied by a calcaneovalgus deformity which resolves spontaneously with time. The bowing itself normally resolves by the 4th birthday, although a residual leg length discrepancy is often apparent at skeletal maturity. The degree of leg discrepancy is thought to be independent of the initial degree of bowing and is typically about 4 cm.

Congenital Vertical Talus (CVT)

Congenital vertical talus or congenital convex pes valgus is a rare condition. The aetiology is unknown but family history is a known risk factor. Half of cases are bilateral and up to half are associated with an underlying genetic or neuromuscular disorder such as myelodysplasias, arthrogryposis or chromosomal abnormalities (Fig. 11.4).

Symptoms and Signs

This presents shortly after birth with a fixed deformity.
Examination findings reveal:

- The foot is in dorsiflexion.
- Medial arch is flat.
- Hindfoot is often in a valgus position and potentially equinus.
- The vertical talus position will result in a convex or "rocker-bottom" shape to the plantar surface of the midfoot.

There are four abnormalities that are always present in a true CVT:

- Irreducible dorsal navicular dislocation.
- Peroneus longus and tibialis posterior displacement such as they act as dorsiflexors.

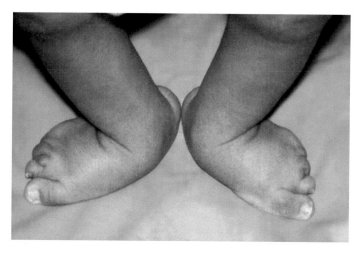

FIGURE 11.4 Bilateral CVT. Note the forefoot valgus and eversion. (Reproduced from Benson et al. *Children's Orthopaedics and Fractures*, 2009, Springer)

- Talo-calcaneal joint subluxation.
- Fixed ankle equinus.

The most common differentials to consider are a calcaneo-valgus or plano-valgus foot, or an oblique talus. A true CVT is distinguished from the aforementioned conditions through the rigid, non-correctable position of the talus. Plantar flexion stress lateral radiographs (the Eyre-Brook view) help determine the position of the talus and it's flexibility relative to the navicular and first ray (Fig. 11.5).

Treatment

The aim of treatment is to restore the bones to their normal anatomical position, correcting the following deformities:

- Talo-navicular dislocation.
- Hindfoot equinus.
- Forefoot eversion.

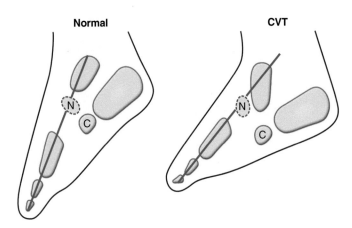

FIGURE 11.5 Diagram demonstrating the plantar-flexion stress lateral radiographs of normal and congenital vertical talus feet. A further key radiographic finding is the fixed dorsal dislocation of the navicular. The navicular is dotted as it is the last bone in the foot to ossify but its position can be determined by drawing a line through the first ray

Non-operative

- Non-operative treatment rarely succeeds in successfully treating CVT and so intervention is normally required.
- Manipulations and serial casting: Manipulation into plantar-flexed and inverted positions form part of the 'reverse Ponseti' method. This method is successful, is the first-line of treatment and is increasing in popularity, although recurrence is an issue. A mini-open reduction of the talo-navicular joint is seen as part of the reverse Ponseti technique, along with any lengthening of involved dorsiflexors and evertors and an Achilles tenotomy, all performed at the end of the casting period.

Surgical Intervention

Surgery is normally performed between the ages of 6 months and 2 years and is usually preceded by serial 'reverse Ponseti' casting. A variety of techniques have been described which include soft tissue releases, lengthening of the dorsolateral tendons (Achilles, peroneals, extensors) and reconstruction of the calcaneonavicular (spring) ligament. Open or mini-open reduction techniques can be combined with soft tissue release to reduce the talus. This often requires maintaining reduction with a K-wire, later removed at 6 weeks. The recurrence rates of major open CVT surgery are often high (between 60 and 100%) and further revision procedures are often needed as child grows older.

Pes Planus

Flatfoot or pes planus is a common cause of parental anxiety, but the majority of cases are benign conditions that require no orthopaedic intervention. A flat foot is a normal part of childhood development and studies show that this is evident in up to 97% of children less than 18 months of age. In some, this can persist into adulthood (Fig. 11.6).

Symptoms and Signs

Although pes planus is typically asymptomatic, some children may complain of arch pain or pre-tibial pain. However, most will present when toddlers once the parents have noticed the shape of the arches.

The key is differentiating between a flexible flat foot and a pathological one, via clinical examination. Examine the patient standing, and look for:

- Flat medial arch.
- Tight tendo Achilles – examine the gastrocsoleus complex with Silverskiold's test.
- Gait pattern and changes in the arch through the stance phase.
- Ask the child to stand on tip toes and observe that the arch is restored, the heel will move from valgus to varus and the tibia externally rotates.

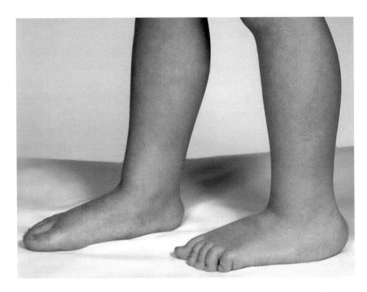

FIGURE 11.6 Pes planus (Reproduced from Benson et al. *Children's Orthopaedics and Fractures*, 2009, Springer)

- A very young child may not be able to stand on tip toes and in this situation, the clinician should dorsiflex the big toe and observe similar changes as seen when standing on tip toes (Jack's test or Hubscher manoeuvre).

A stiff or rigid flat foot or hindfoot is an abnormal sign and should prompt further investigation. Examine muscle bulk and rigidity in the lower limbs, as this could be the presenting sign of an underlying neuromuscular condition. A flexible flatfoot may be associated with hypermobility so it is important to look for this at this stage.

Differential Diagnosis

- Vertical Talus: Causes a flat medial arch but other signs, such as fixed dorsiflexion, will be present.
- Postural defects: Results in a compensatory flat-foot.

- Tendo Achilles tightness/contracture: Cause eversion of the foot and the foot will compensate by going into valgus.
- Tarsal coalition: An abnormal connection between two or more tarsal bones. The coalitions restrict the subtalar joint and the distal joints. A flat medial arch is a compensatory mechanism for the deformity.

  - Connections are fibrous (syndesmosis), cartilaginous (synchondrosis) or osseous (synostosis).
  - Most commonly present in adolescence with a painful, flat foot.
  - Calcaneo-navicular coalition is the most common type but talo-calcaneal coalitions are also seen.
  - May include peroneal spasm resulting in calf pain, and is therefore also described as peroneal spastic flat-foot.
  - Radiographs may reveal:

    - 'Anteater's nose' sign is seen in calcaneo-navicular coalitions and is best seen on the lateral X-ray of the foot.
    - A calcenao-navicular bar may be seen on 45° oblique view X-ray of the foot (Fig. 11.7).
    - 'C sign' seen in talo-calcaneal coalitions and is best seen on the lateral X-ray of the ankle (Fig. 11.8).
    - In most cases CT or MRI scan will be helpful to confirm the diagnosis and exclude other coalitions in the foot.

Treatment

An asymptomatic flexible flat foot should be considered a normal variant. In the neurologically normal patient, no treatment is required. Studies have shown that orthotics or specialist inserts do not alter the natural history of the condition.

The symptomatic flat foot may benefit from tendo Achilles stretching if a tight tendon is felt to be a contributing factor. Surgery is generally avoided but options include calcaneal osteotomies and other interventions to alter column length, as described by Evans.

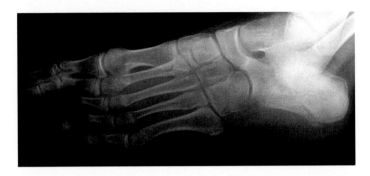

FIGURE 11.7 Oblique X-ray of foot demonstrating a calcaneo-navicular coalition

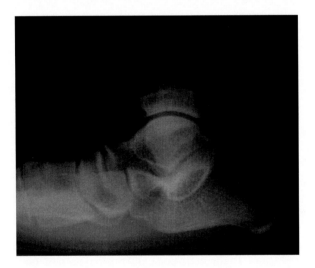

FIGURE 11.8 'C sign' of a talo-calcaneal coalition

Tarsal coalition can be a difficult condition to treat.

- Non-operative: Immobilisation in a walking plaster for up to 6 weeks. Can be combined with a manipulation under anaesthesia or guided injection of local anaesthetic or steroid. Prolonged splinting with inserts or an orthosis may be required for up to 6 months.

- Surgical: Excision of a calcaneonavicular bar is successful if there is no secondary degenerative change elsewhere or any other associated coalitions in the same foot. Talocalcaneal coalitions respond less well to surgery and a realignment calcaneal osteotomy or a delayed triple arthrodesis may be preferred if symptoms persist.

Flat feet

- Considered a normal variant if flexible and neurologically normal.
- Look for tarsal coalition in the stiff foot.
- Secondary degenerative joint may be the true source of pain.

Pes Cavus

A cavus foot is one with an abnormal elevation of the medial arch that does not reduce on weight bearing. The foot can be considered a tripod, the points of contact being the first metatarsal head, the fifth metatarsal head and the heel. Elevation of the medial arch, or a cavus deformity, can be caused by a plantar-flexed first ray which forces the mid-foot up and into varus and consequentially the hindfoot into varus. This is a so-called forefoot driven cavo-varus. Conversely, in hindfoot driven pathologies, the hindfoot (i.e. heel) is either already in varus or can not evert, and the forefoot secondarily plantar flexes.

The causes of a cavus foot are summarised in Table 11.2. Neurological abnormalities leading to muscle imbalances are responsible for 2/3 of diagnoses. In such cases, imbalanced action between agonistic and antagonistic muscles brings about the deformity.

- The powerful peroneus longus muscle overcomes the weaker tibialis anterior to cause the first MTP to plantarflex and the high arch to manifest.
- The posterior tibialis muscle pulls harder than the weak peroneus brevis, causing forefoot adduction and a varus deformity of the hindfoot.

TABLE 11.2 Causes of a cavus foot, classified as per the anatomical cause and aetiology

Classification as per anatomical cause	
Forefoot driven causes	**Hindfoot driven causes**
Peroneus longus hyperactivity	Clubfoot
Tight gastrocnemius	Trauma
	Tarsal coalition
	Deep posterior compartment scarring
Aetiology	
Neuromuscular	Muscle – Muscular dystrophy Nerves – Charcot-Marie-Tooth, intraspinal tumour, polyneuritis, spinal dysraphism Anterior horn spinal cord – Polio, syringomyelia, tumours, muscular atrophy, spinal dysraphism Long tract/central nervous system – Friedreich's ataxia, Roussy-Levy syndrome, cerebellar diseases, cerebral palsy
Congenital	Idiopathic clubfoot Arthrogryposis
Traumatic	Residuals of compartment syndrome Crush injuries Burns Malunion of foot fractures

- Unopposed action of the ankle dorsiflexors, due to a weak triceps surae, further leads to an abnormal position of the calcaneum relative to the first ray.
- Claw or cock up deformities of the toes are further caused by contraction of the small intrinsic muscle and the long extensors to the toes. With the forefoot valgus and the hindfoot varus, instability of the ankle may ensue given the increased stress placed on the lateral ankle ligaments.

Patients typically present in later childhood. When evaluating a child with pes cavus, the history and examination must focus on determining the cause of the deformity and must include a full neurological examination. The examination should include a Coleman Block Test, which assesses the flexibility of the hindfoot. If the varus is corrected when standing on the block, the pathology is likely forefoot driven and hence correction of the forefoot should correct the cavus. Conversely, a rigid varus hindfoot on the block suggests hindfoot driven pathology (Fig. 11.9).

Pes cavus can be treated by non-operative or operative means.

Non-operative

The use of orthoses and foot wear modification is reserved for the milder forms where there is no significant imbalance. Although they do not alter the natural progression of the deformity they are able to provide milder support.

Operative

A variety of surgical options are available to the surgeon and they depend on a series of factors.

Surgical options include:

- **Plantar fascia release:** The plantar fascia normally is contracted and needs to be released. Milder deformities may be treated with releases alone or they may be used to augment other procedures.
- **Midtarsal osteotomy:** A wedge of bone is excised from the cuboid and cuneiforms.

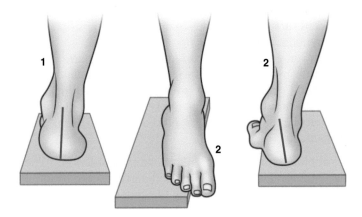

FIGURE 11.9 The Coleman Block Test. The normal hindfoot is in approximately 5° of valgus. When assessing a cavus foot from behind (*1*), the hindfoot will be in varus and more toes will be visible medially compared to the normal foot (opposite of the too many toes sign). If the varus is corrected when the patient stands on the block (*2*), the deformity is said to be 'forefoot driven'. Conversely, if the deformity is not corrected the deformity is considered to be driven by the hindfoot

- **First metatarsal extension osteotomy:** Normally a dorsally based osteotomy, designed to avoid the proximal physis.
- **Calcaneal osteotomy:** Particularly in the older child with a hindfoot deformity, a calcaneal valgus displacement or lateral wedge osteotomy may be performed.
- **Tendon transfers:** Various tendon transfers are possible, and the choice largely depends on the pathology, age and severity of the deformity.

Factors that affect decision-making include:

- **Child age:** Broadly speaking, the younger child may get away with soft tissue procedures and tendon transfers alone, whereas the older child is more likely to require bony procedures.

- **Flexibility or rigidity:** The more rigid the deformity, the greater the need for bony procedures to augment soft tissue procedures. In cases where the hind foot is flexible, correction of the forefoot deformity may suffice. If the hindfoot varus is being driven by a rigid hindfoot, then correction of it (for example a calcaneal osteotomy) may be required.
- **Aetiology of the lesion:** Particularly in the case of the neurological causes, determining the instigating abnormality will aid in determining treatment, for example, which tendon transfers to perform. Similarly, removing the implicated driving force of the cavus may well treat the secondary deformity, for example lengthening a contracted Achille's tendon in a CP patient whose deformity is driven by a tight gastrocsoleus complex.

Accessory Navicular

The accessory navicular is a benign ossicle, which can be considered a normal variant, present in up to 12% of children. Three types exist:

Type 1: A small sesmoid type ossicle which resides in the tibialis posterior tendon.

Type 2: A larger lesion (around 1 cm in diameter) that is joined to the navicular by a cartilaginous bridge.

Type 3: A complete bony enlargement of the navicular.

Symptoms often develop in later childhood and are often due to overuse, stress, shoes or trauma, resulting form microfractures at the synchondrosis, or from disruption of the posterior tibialis tendon. The chief complaint is medial arch pain. The symptoms can be controlled with activity modification, which may require initial immobilisation in plaster for a short period of time. If symptoms persist, surgical excision can be performed. Type 1 lesions rarely require operative intervention.

Juvenile Hallux Valgus

Hallux valgus is rare in young children and when present, it can be associated with conditions such as Apert's Syndrome. Usually, hallux valgus will present in adolescence. It is more common in girls, is often bilateral, there may be evidence of ligamentous laxity and there is often a positive family history. Historically this has been linked with poorly fitting footwear but current ideas do not support this theory. Initial treatment involves modification to wide-fitting footwear to alleviate symptoms rather than prevent progression. If the deformity is persistent and symptomatic, then surgery can be considered. This is best delayed until skeletal maturity because of the risk of recurrence. Surgery is recommended in patients with a hallux valgus angle of >20° and an intermetatarsal angle of >15°. Procedures are similar to adults and complications include recurrence and overcorrection.

Toe Abnormalities

- Syndactyly: This is a congenital fusion of the toes, most commonly the second and third, and is associated with underlying genetic conditions such at Down's syndrome. This can be a soft tissue fusion (simple) or bony (complex). Simple syndactyly is often observed with digital release indicated in complex deformities.
- Polydactyly: Extra digits are common laterally (post-axial) but can occur both centrally and medially (pre-axial). These are associated with a positive family history or an underlying tibial hemimelia. If the digit is well aligned, they can be observed. Small rudimentary digits can be ligated at birth. If the toe is malaligned or causing excess widening of the foot, it can be surgically excised. This is best performed at 9–12 months of age.
- Oligodactyly: This congenital absence of one or more toes may be associated with other toe abnormalities, tarsal coalitions or fibular hemimelia. There is usually no limitation in function and no treatment is required.

- Overlapping toe: This is most common in the fifth toe and is often bilateral. It can interfere with footwear. First line treatments include neighbour strapping and passive stretches. If it continues to be symptomatic, surgical options include the release of EDL alone or in combination with a dorsal capsulotomy and syndactilisation using a McFarland's Procedure. Furthermore, Butler and Cockin described a double V-Y plasty on the sole and dorsum of the foot. The two are joined so that the deformity is not only released, but pulled plantigrade. Bony procedures or even amputation of the fifth toe are reserved as salvage procedures and last resorts.
- Congenital curly toe: This usually involves the lateral three toes and if often bilateral. Clinically there is a flexion and varus at the interphalangeal joint secondary to contractures of FDL of FDB. There is usually no limitation in function and no treatment is required in the vast majority as spontaneous resolution is the norm. Surgical options include tenotomy of the involved tendons if the deformities do not correct by the age of 3.
- Congenital hallux varus: Otherwise described as atavistic great toe, this deformity presents after walking with a varus deformity at the metatarsophalangeal joint of the big toe. It is associated with polydactyly. Most deformities correct with age and treatment is rarely indicated. In persistent and symptomatic cases, abductor hallucis release is the treatment of choice.

Key References

Evans AM, Rome K. A Cochrane review of the evidence for non-surgical interventions for flexible pediatric flat feet. Eur J Phys Rehabil Med. 2011;47(1):69–89.

Wright J, Coggings D, Maizen C, Ramachandran M. Reverse Ponseti-type treatment for children with congenital vertical talus: comparison between idiopathic and teratological patients. Bone Joint J. 2014;96-B(2):274–8.

Schwend RM, Drennan JC. Cavus foot deformity in children. J Am Acad Orthop Surg. 2003;11(3):201–11.

Chapter 12
Congenital Talipes Equinovarus (Clubfoot)

Joanna Thomas and Matthew Barry

Definition

Congential talipes equinovarus (CTEV) is a congenital disorder affecting the foot which presents at birth with the hindfoot in equinus and varus, the midfoot in adduction and often cavus and the forefoot adducted.

Aetiology and Epidemiology

This has been ascribed to a combination of environmental and genetic factors.

J. Thomas, MSc, FRCS (Tr&Orth)
T&O SpR Royal London Rotation, London, UK

M. Barry, MS, FRCS (Orth) (✉)
Paediatric and Young Adult Orthopaedic Unit,
The Royal London and The London Children's Hospitals,
Barts Health NHS Trust, London, UK
e-mail: matthew.barry@bartshealth.nhs.uk

N.A. Aresti et al. (eds.), *Paediatric Orthopaedics in Clinical Practice*, In Clinical Practice, DOI 10.1007/978-1-4471-6769-3_12, © Springer-Verlag London 2016

The evidence for a genetic influence includes:

- Family history:
  - 25% of patients with isolated clubfoot will have a positive family history.
  - A sibling of a child with a clubfoot has a 2–4% chance of also being affected.
  - Twin studies demonstrating monozygotic twins have a much higher rate of both children being affected (33%) as opposed to dizygotic twins (3%).
  - Being male is a risk factor.

- Race preponderance, with an incidence of 0.39 per 1000 in Chinese, 1.2 per 1000 live births in Caucasians and 6.9 per 1000 in Polynesians, although it is currently believed that CTEV may be of similar incidence in all ethnic groups and geographies.

Evidence in support of environmental influences include:

- Maternal smoking increases the risk of clubfoot by an odds ratio of approximately 1.3.
- Early amniocentesis ($11^{+0} \rightarrow 12^{+6}$ weeks) may carry increased risk of clubfoot, whereas mid-trimester amniocentesis ($15^{+0} \rightarrow 16^{+6}$ gestational weeks) was found to carry a risk equal to that of the general population. This would suggest a critical point in development during the first trimester of pregnancy.
- Low birth weight may carry an increased risk of clubfoot.

The above evidence suggests the development of clubfoot follows a complex inheritance pattern that is influenced by several environmental factors. Although it is not a sex-linked disorder, gender has an influence. This suggests females require a higher load of abnormal genes to develop a clubfoot, and therefore in turn means they are more likely to pass abnormal genes on. This is known as the 'Carter effect'.

Diagnosis

The diagnosis is often made at birth by observing the position of the foot (Fig. 12.1). It is important to differentiate from the relatively common calcaneovalgus foot and the rare congenital vertical talus (Chap. 11). A defining difference is the inability to dorsiflex a clubfoot child's ankle past neutral. When the child is assessed for the first time in clinic, it is important to not only examine the foot, but also the hips and the base of the spine as well.

The use of ultrasound in clubfoot is also increasing. Its use prenatally to diagnose the condition intrauterine is now well established (Fig. 12.2).

Radiographic analysis can be obtained to differentiate from a vertical talus, although X-rays are less commonly used for diagnosis and treatment currently (Fig. 12.3).

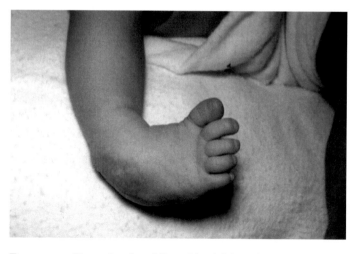

FIGURE 12.1 Example of an idiopathic clubfoot deformity – this is the same child as Fig. 12.2

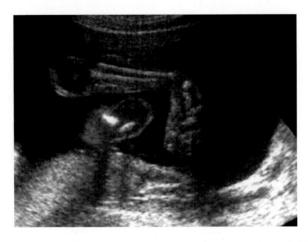

FIGURE 12.2 An antenatal ultrasound scan demonstrating a clubfoot

On The AP view, the following observations can be made:

1. Lines drawn through the long axis of the calcaneum and talus will give a talo-calcaneal (Kite) angle of less than 20° (in a normal foot this would be between 20 and 40°). This is known as " parallelism" of the talus and calcaneum.
2. Lines are drawn down the long axis of the first meta-tarsal and the talus. In a foot with talipes the angle is "negative" or in adduction; in a normal foot, it is in slight abduction – 30°.
3. There is also medial displacement of the cuboid ossification centre.

On the lateral radiograph, lines are drawn through the long axis of the talus and the inferior margin of the calcaneum – in a patient with CTEV, the angle is less than 25°.

Grading

The Pirani grading system is helpful to monitor initial treatment and early progress, and is the most commonly employed clinically (Table 12.1). It involves scoring based on six clinical

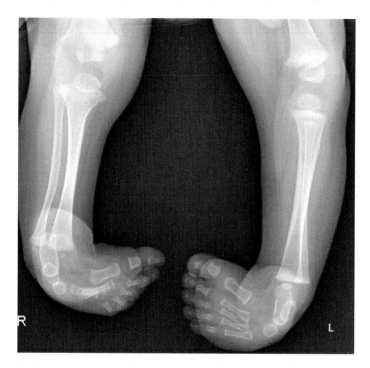

FIGURE 12.3 Radiograph of the lower limbs in a patient with bilateral clubfoot deformity

signs of contracture with 0 being no abnormality, 0.5 mild abnormality and 1 severe abnormality.

The areas assessed are:

The hindfoot:

1. Severity of the posterior crease.
2. Emptiness of the heel pad.
3. Rigidity of the equinus.

In the midfoot:

1. Curvature of the lateral border of the foot.
2. Severity of the medial crease.
3. Position of the lateral head of the talus.

The other well known scoring system, the Dimeglio system, scores four essential parameters based on severity and four "pejorative elements", but this system is rarely used in contemporary treatment.

Management

Although both operative and non-operative methods have been employed in the treatment of clubfoot, the mainstay of management is now based around non-operative methods, in particular the Ponseti method. It involves serial casting with or without an Achilles tenotomy, followed by the use of 'boots and bars'. The French functional physiotherapy method also has good results, although it is a far more intensive treatment regimen.

The manoeuvres, which precede serial casting, target specific elements of the clubfoot deformity. The order in which they are performed is important, following the acronym CAVE (cavus, adductus, varus, equinus) (Fig. 12.4).

The first manoeuvre to correct the deformity is to align the first ray with the rest of the metatarsals in order to correct the cavus. This is followed by casting with lateral pressure on

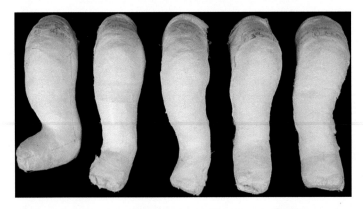

FIGURE 12.4 Examples of plaster casts that follow the Ponseti regimen (Reproduced from Benson et al. *Children's Orthopaedics and Fractures*, 2009)

the talar head, in order to correct the forefoot adductus and hind-foot varus. At this point, an Achilles tenotomy is performed in the majority ($\approx$90%), after which the equinus is corrected in the final cast.

Each time full above knee casts are used and changed every 1 to 2 weeks. After 6–8 weeks of treatment with casting, Denis-Browne 'boots and bars' are used up to 4 years. They are used 23/24 h a day (but can be removed for washing) for the first 3 months. They can reduce down to night-time and nap-times for the following 2–3 years.

There is a relapse rate, which is why it is imperative to continue to follow these children in a clinic. They should be examined every 6 months until the age of 5 years, then can go to yearly examinations.

If a recurrence occurs, it can be identified by tightening of the tendo-Achilles, which will become apparent when examining dorsiflexion of the ankle joint with the leg extended and with the knee flexed. On assessing their gait, initial contact will be with the lateral border of the foot. They will weight transfer on the lateral border of their foot in the stance phase and start to develop dynamic supination through the swing phase as they dorsiflex the foot prior to initial contact (due to activation of tibialis anterior without opposition from inactive peroneals).

Depending on the age of the patient, it is advisable to try repeat serial casting or progress to surgical management.

Surgical Management

If the recurrence is mild and the child is older than three, it may be that only a lateral tibialis anterior tendon transfer to the lateral cuneiform is needed, along with a minor posterior release to correct the hindfoot.

Surgical release for severe, recurrent deformity that responds poorly to Ponseti is usually delayed until at least 6–9 months of age. It is very important to preserve the neurovascular structures of the foot. Two main approaches have been described – a Cincinnati incision or an oblique Turco incision, the latter being preferred for cosmesis. Numerous procedures have been described but the main aim is to release the posterior and medial structures.

The Achilles tendon needs to be lengthened by Z-lengthening, and the calcaneofibular ligament and posterior talofibular ligament should be released. Then the structures behind the medial malleous: tibialis posterior tendon, flexor digitorum longus and flexor hallucis longus are lengthened as needed, the superficial deltoid is released as is the tibiotalar, subtalar and tibionavicular joint capsules. The foot may be held in place with K-wires (although metalwork is best avoided if possible), followed by above knee casting.

Late Presentation

Late presentation is common amongst developing countries, although the advent of large scale Ponseti programmes has seen rates reduce globally. Conservative treatment is still possible, and indeed has been documented as being successful even in adults (18 year olds). Surgery however is more likely. If the child is aged between 3 and 10 years, a medial opening osteotomy or a lateral closing wedge osteotomy may be performed to correct the midfoot deformity.

In those presenting very late, i.e. older than 8, a primary triple arthrodesis remains a viable option. A talectomy may occasionally be the only course of management, particularly in the insensate foot.

Synopsis

CTEV is a congenital foot deformity with hindfoot equinus and varus, along with midfoot varus and forefoot adductus. Its incidence is 1.44 per 1000 live births. The aetiology includes environmental and genetic factors (32.5% of both siblings affected in monozygotic twins) and it is twice as common in boys than girls. CTEV is most commonly classified clinically using the Pirani scoring system (Table 12.1). The mainstay of treatment is

TABLE 12.1 Table depicting the Pirani scoring system

HFCS	PC	The severity of the posterior crease	0	Multiple fine creases
Hindfoot contracture score			0.5	One or two deep creases
		Foot held in maximal correction	1	Deep creases change the contour of the arch
	EH	The emptiness of the heel	0	Tuberosity of calcaneus easily palpable
		Foot held in maximal correction	0.5	Tuberosity of calcaneus more difficult to palpate
			1	Tuberosity of calcaneus not palpable
	RE	Rigidity of equinus	0	Ankle dorsiflexes fully
		Knee extended, ankle maximally corrected	0.5	Ankle dorsiflexes to 'neutral' angle between lateral border of foot and leg ≤90°
			1	Ankle dorsiflexion severely limited – fixed equinus. angle between lateral border of foot and leg >90°

(continued)

TABLE 12.1 (continued)

MFCS	MC	Severity of the medial crease		
Midfoot contracture score			0	Multiple fine creases
		Foot held in maximal correction	0.5	One or two deep creases
			1	Deep creases change the contour of the arch
	LHT	Palpation of the lateral part of the head of the talus	0	Navicular completely reduces, lateral talar head cannot be felt
		Forefoot held fully abducted	0.5	Navicular partially reduces, lateral talar head less palpable
			1	Navicular does not reduce, lateral talar head easily felt
	CLB	The curvature of the lateral border	0	Straight border
			0.5	Mild curve of lateral border distally
			1	Lateral border curves at calcaneo-cuboid joint

non-operative, most often with Ponseti serial casting. The surgical options that are employed, mainly in the resistant, relapsing or late presenting foot, include surgical releases, lengthening of the tendo-Achilles and ligaments behind the medial malleolus and posterior medial joint capsules, along with tendon transfers and osteotomies.

Key References

Jowett CR, Morcuende JA, Ramachandran M. Management of congenital talipes equinovarus using the Ponseti method A SYSTEMATIC REVIEW. J Bone Joint Surg. 2011;93(9):1160–4.
Barry M. Prenatal assessment of foot deformity. Early Human Dev 2005;81:793–6.

Chapter 13
Lower Limb Alignment and Leg Length Discrepancy

Charlie Jowett and Matthew Barry

Definition

Leg length discrepancy (LLD) is a condition of unequal lengths of the lower limbs. It can be subdivided into the following categories:

- Anatomical LLD – A deformity leading to an LLD may be due to a combination of a reduction in bone length and by angular deformity.
- Functional LLD – Typically a contracture of the lower limb muscles will cause a functional discrepancy. A fixed pelvic obliquity due to a deformity of the lumbar spine (i.e. scoliosis) may similarly lead to a functional pattern.

C. Jowett, FRCS (Tr&Orth)
T&O SpR Royal London Rotation, London, UK

M. Barry, MS, FRCS (Orth) (✉)
Paediatric and Young Adult Orthopaedic Unit,
The Royal London and The London Children's Hospitals,
Barts Health NHS Trust, London, UK
e-mail: matthew.barry@bartshealth.nhs.uk

N.A. Aresti et al. (eds.), *Paediatric Orthopaedics in Clinical Practice*, In Clinical Practice, DOI 10.1007/978-1-4471-6769-3_13, © Springer-Verlag London 2016

Symptoms and Signs

Children typically compensate for LLD by altering their pelvic obliquity (particularly when the LLD is <2 cm), flexing their knee on the longer side or walking with an equinus foot on the shorter side, or on tiptoe.

The body is able to compensate for an LLD of less than 2 cm. Greater differences in leg length inequality will cause postural imbalance in standing and an uneven gait, which can lead to heightened stresses on the longer of the two legs and spinal imbalance.

There is a higher prevalence of back pain when there is a LLD of greater than 15 mm, in the order of 5.3× greater than the general population. Arthritic changes are more common with an LLD. It is more common in the hip (84%) and knee of the longer leg.

Clinical Assessment

It is important to distinguish between a *true* and *apparent* LLD and to determine whether the deformity originates above or below the knee. It is important also to bear in mind that patients may have elements of both and that they will compensate for a deformity by altering their function.

Two main methods may be used to assess LLD:

- Blocks – incremental blocks will allow visual assessment of correction of pelvic and spinal alignment.
- Tape measurement – leg lengths are measured in the supine position, from either the xiphisternum (apparent) or ASIS (real) to the medial malleolus of the ankle.

To specifically examine the origin of the shortening and whether there is true or apparent discrepancy, flex both knees with the heels remaining on the couch at the same level. Tibial shortening causes the knee to lie lower than the unaffected side. Femoral shortening causes the knee to adopt a more proximal position. In the case of the later (femoral shortening), the degree of the deformity may be calculated in relation to the greater trochanter. This can be deduced from Bryant's triangle, Nelaton's line and Schoemaker's line (Fig. 13.1).

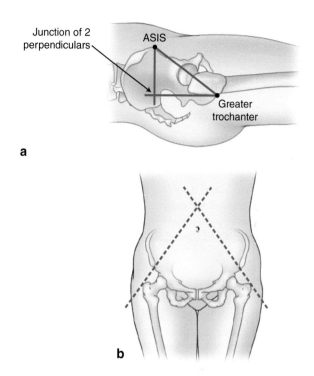

FIGURE 13.1 Bryant's triangle (**a**) helps differentiate between supra- and infratrochanteric shortening of the femur. A *line* is drawn from the ASIS (A) to the tip of the greater trochanter (B). *Horizontal and vertical lines* are drawn as demonstrated, intersecting at point (C), forming the triangle. The distance between points B&C correlate to the femoral neck, and comparison with the contralateral side may indicate shortening. Nelaton's line runs from the ASIS to the ischial tuberosity. The greater trochanter should just touch the line. Proximal migration of the trochanter would suggest supratrochanteric shortening. Finally, Shoemaker's line (**b**) also runs from the greater trochanter to the ASIS and beyond towards the abdomen. Both Shoemaker's lines should intersect at or above the umbilicus in the midline. If they cross below, supratrochanteric shortening should be assumed

Finally the patient's gait must be observed. If there is a significant discrepancy, they will have a short leg gait.

Epidemiology

LLD's are relatively common, with a reported prevalence of 90% in normal adults with a mean inequality of 5.2 mm. LLD greater than 20 mm affects 1 in 1,000 people.

Aetiology

The aetiology of a pathological leg length discrepancy can be congenital acquired, and may shorten the limb or lengthen it. In cases of congenital defects, LLD can be calculated and predicted more easily as growth remains proportional. This is not the case in acquired disorders.

Limb Alignment

Limb deformities can happen in all planes. Normally up until the age of two there is a prevalence for physiological genu varum (bowlegs), between the ages of three and six children develop genu valgum (knock knees). This is physiological up to the age of eight or ten and persists to a mild degree in many adults (see Chap. 1) (Fig. 13.2). The onset or persistence of angular deformities after the age of 6 should be viewed with suspicion. Asymmetrical deformities and those associated with pain should be investigated.

Causes of a Shortened Limb

A summary of the different aetiologies of malalignment is summarised in Table 13.1.

Congenital

The majority of congenital limb deficiencies occur sporadically. Three main forms of congenital shortening of the lower limb exist:

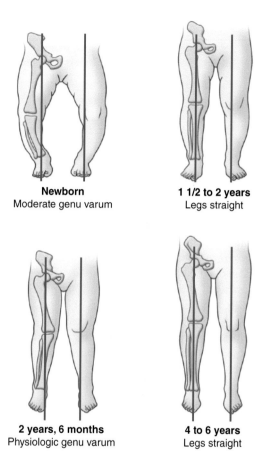

Newborn
Moderate genu varum

1 1/2 to 2 years
Legs straight

2 years, 6 months
Physiologic genu varum

4 to 6 years
Legs straight

FIGURE 13.2 Normal evolution of coronal alignment of the lower limbs

- Congenital femoral deficiency.
  - This includes idiopathic coxa vara (see Chap. 9), congenital short femur and proximal femoral focal deficiency (PFFD).
  - Of the latter two, congenital short femur is the milder form with an average growth retardation of about 10%. PFFD is a developmental defect of the proximal femur and ranges from hypoplasia of the proximal femur to

TABLE 13.1 Aetiology of lower limb malalignment

Cause	Genu valgum	Genu varum
Congenital	Fibular hemimelia Skeletal dysplasia	Tibial hemimelia Skeletal dysplasia
Trauma	Partial physeal arrest	Partial physeal arrest
Arthritis	Juvenile RA	
Infection	Partial growth arrest	Partial growth arrest
Metabolic	Rickets	Rickets
Others		Blount's disease

Adapted from *Childrens orthopaedics and fractures* by Benson et al., 2009, Springer

  complete absence of the proximal end. In truth, they are not separate disorders but a continuum of a spectrum of disorders.
  – The cause of this is unknown and it can be associated with other anomalies in the limbs and face.
  – In 1969 Aitken developed a classification (A–D), which describes the appearance of the acetabulum with reference to the femoral head and the increasing coxa vara that increases with severity.

• Congenital fibular deficiency (Fig. 13.3).

  – It is the most common of the lower limb congenital deficiencies.
  – It similarly includes a spectrum of deformities from mild shortening of the tibia and fibula to complete absence with tibial shortening and bowing along with foot deformity.
  – Clinically the patient may have anteriomedial bowing of the tibia and a dimple over the skin at the apex of the tibial bow. The foot is normally in an equinovalgus position.
  – It is associated with congenital femoral deficiency, cruciate ligament deficiency, tarsal coalition and absent lateral rays.

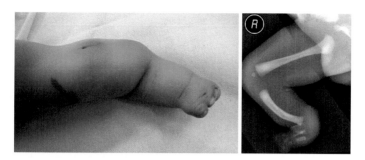

FIGURE 13.3 Congenital fibula deficiency clinical photograph and X-ray

- Congenital tibial deficiency.

  - This is the rarest of the congenital abnormalities described, and may also be seen at varying degrees of severity.
  - The typical appearance is that of an anterolateral bowed tibia. The knee is normally in varus with a prominent fibula head. The foot is in equinovarus and it may show medial duplication/polydactyly.

- Other congenital causes to be aware of include developmental dysplasia of the hip (Figs. 13.4), Ollier's disease and CTEV.

Acquired

Acquired causes of leg shortening include:

- Infection/Inflammation.

  - Including osteomyelitis (metaphyseal) and septic arthritis (with growth plate damage).

- Tumour.

  - Including osteochondromas, Wilm's tumour and can be a complication of radiation treatment.

FIGURE 13.4 Apparent leg length discrepancy due to DDH and dislocated hip

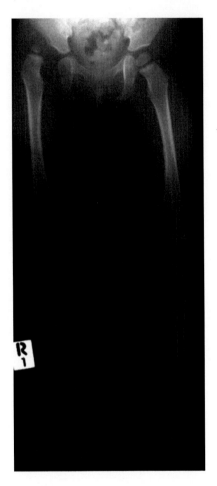

- Neurological diseases.
  - Including poliomyelitis, myelomeningocele and contractures due to cerebral palsy.
- Post traumatic.
  - Can be following growth arrest from a traumatic injury or a slipped upper femoral epiphysis.

Calculating Growth Rate

Various methods have been described which predict the remaining growth of bone and prediction of progression of a deformity in the limbs.

Bone age:

Various systems have been used. The atlas of Greulich and Pyle uses gender specific details of the radiograph of the left hand to determine bone age. The Tanner and Whitehouse system uses 20 indicators on the AP hand radiograph but is very time consuming.

Methods for predicting future LLD:

Arithmetic method: Introduced by White and Menelaus. The rate of leg growth is 56% from the femur, 4 mm a year proximally and 9 mm/year distally. The growth is 46% from the tibia, 6 mm/year proximally and 4 mm/year distally. Leg length discrepancy can be calculated assuming that girls stop growing at 14 and boys at 16 years of age. However this method does not take into account growth spurts.

Growth remaining method: Introduced by Green and Anderson who reviewed 100 children from Boston (50% of which had polio affecting one leg). They correlated growth to skeletal matruity with the Greulich and Pyle bone age atlas, and found the accuracy of assessing growth inhibition improved over 3–4 years of age.

Straight line method: Moseley derived this method from the Green and Anderson data/tables from which they used more complicated straight line tables.

Paley's multiplier method: This method is used to predict adult height, bone length and timing of epiphysiodesis. It is derived from an arithmetic formula, itself derived from the Green and Anderson growth charts and compared with multipliers from 19 other databases. It is the only method that enables calculation of upper limb discrepancies.

All these methods are valid only when there is constant inhibition of the short limb.

Investigations

Radiological Investigations

Radiography is the gold standard for LLD measurement and will display any associated joint or bone deformity. In particular, the following may be sought:

- Standing long leg alignment radiographs (Figs. 13.5) – These films allow the leg length, foot height and magnitude of shortening to be calculated precisely. This method uses extra long film cassettes (90 cm in most European countries), providing images of the entire lower extremity including the foot and pelvis. A magnification film should be used.
- Orthoroentgenogram – These images are taken with the patient lying supine with a full scale between the patient's legs on the table. Three separate images are taken with the central ray centred over the hip, knee and ankle respectively. These images allow the true length of the femur and tibia to be calculated. However this method does not provide information on functional LLD, pelvic obliquity and foot height.
- Teleroentgenogram – This involves a single 3-foot radiograph taken of the lower extremities. Entire bones are shown so malalignment or lesions in the bone will be apparent. The disadvantage is that the film is distorted by magnification at the upper and lower ends of the film.

Management of Leg Length Discrepancy

The key to treatment is to predict what the discrepancy is at maturity. The aims of treatment are to level the pelvis and avoid secondary problems such as low back pain and

FIGURE 13.5 Long leg view radio-graph of a LLD with a short tibia

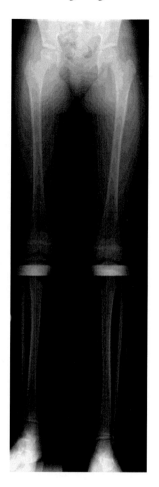

secondary osteoarthritis. Surgical management depends on age, pathology, severity, projected height at the end of growth and associated deformities.

No treatment is generally required in adults with a discrepancy of less than 2 cm unless symptomatic. If the discrepancy is greater than 2 cm, a shoe raise can be used.

Surgical Limb Equalisation

Leg Shortening

In a child of normal height at maturation and an anticipated discrepancy of 2–5 cm, shortening should be the method of choice. Several options exist:

Epiphysiodesis – This is surgical interruption of the growth of the longer leg's physis/es and can be used for permanent growth arrest. Epiphysiodesis of the distal femoral epiphysis is used to shorten the femur, and that of the proximal tibial and fibula physis is used to shorten the tibia and fibula.

Permanent epiphysiodesis should be timed to take account of the skeletal age of the child and the anticipated cessation of growth – too soon and the contralateral limb will end up too long and too late, there will not be sufficient time to correct the discrepancy before skeletal maturity. A number of methods have been described:

- Phemister technique – a large diameter core of bone and physis removed, rotated though 90° and re-inserted.
- Percutaneous drilling across the physis under X-ray control, effectively destroying the growth plate (this is the most commonly employed technique) (Fig. 13.3).
- Stapling – staples are placed across the physis on both the medial and lateral aspects.
- Lag screws – screws are placed across the physis from the metaphysis into the epiphysis.
- Guided growth plates – these two hole plates are more commonly used on one side to correct angular deformity but can be placed on both sides to produce a growth arrest, similar to the use of staples.

Leg Lengthening

Limb lengthening is achieved using distraction osteotomies. An osteotomy is accompanied by a mechanical device, which should:

- Allow for lengthening.
- Permit simultaneous accurate correction of deformities in all planes.
- Be user friendly.
- Provide stability for bone regeneration.

This is achieved by using either:

- An extra-medullary device or external fixator – e.g. a 'Taylor Spatial Frame' or an 'Ilizarov' ring fixator (see below).
- An intramedullary (IM) device – e.g. an IM nail.
- A combination of both – using a nail along with an Ilizarov frame, for example, will speed up the healing process.

Osteotomies heal much the same as fractures do i.e. a haematoma collects, followed by soft and hard callus formation and remodelling. Using a low energy and minimally invasive osteotomy (corticotomy) aids the biological process by preserving the blood supply and causing less damage to soft tissues and bone marrow. This can be achieved with a Gigli saw or the DeBastiani technique.

The optimal rate of bone lengthening is 1 mm per day and best achieved in increments of 0.25 mm. After the desired lengthening has been achieved, the external fixator is left until full consolidation is evident. This consolidation phase is often twice as long as the lengthening phase. Up to 20% of bone length can be safely lengthened.

Mechanical Devices for Leg Lengthening

The Ilizarov Ring Fixator

The device is a circular external fixator named after Gavril Abramovich Ilizarov from Kurgan, Siberia. Tensioned Kirschner wires are fixed to the ring and crossed within the bone. Two wires are used at each level and for maximum stability should cross at right angles. Wires should only be placed in anatomical safe zones. The rings are connected by threaded rods and allow correction of the deformity. The advantages of wires are they can be placed in tight spots, permit micromotion in axial loading and stable fixation in osteoporotic bone.

Hexapod Frame

A hexapod system, such as the Taylor Spatial Frame, consists of two rings with six telescope struts. By adjusting only strut length, one ring can be repositioned in relation to the other. A hexapod fixator is capable of correcting 6 axes of deformity guided by a web based software programme. The hexapod frame may be easier to handle than the conventional Ilizarov fixator, especially for rotational and translational deformities, and patients find it easier to use.

Intramedullary Bone Lengthening

Patients often prefer to undergo limb lengthening that does not involve the use of external fixators as external devices severely limit every day activities. Various lengthening intramedullary devices have been designed which can be used if the medullary cavity is wide enough and the patient is approaching skeletal maturity. An example of a lengthening nail is the Precice® nail.

Complications in Limb Lengthening

Several complications may occur when lengthening LLDs. Proper pin site care is essential otherwise infections develop. These may be significantly painful and may lead to local or systemic sepsis. Severe stiffness and dislocation of joints above and below may become apparent. Equinus deformities may develop hence support for the foot during distraction may be of benefit. During lengthening and after removal of the external fixator, fractures may occur. If the bone is dysplastic or there are poor bone regenerative properties, the lengthened bone may be protected by insertion of a K wire.

Large Leg Length Discrepancies

If the anticipated LLD is more than 25 cm at maturity, equalisation by surgery is not advisable by repeated operations; treatment should be orientated to maintaining a good function during childhood and early amputation should be considered. Modern prosthetic technology increasingly provides nearly normal function and quality of life and prostheses are normally well tolerated.

Key References

Knutson GA. Anatomical and functional leg length inequality: a review and recommendation for clinical decision making. Chiropr Osteopat. 2005;13:11.

Tallroth K, Yilkoski M, Lamminem H, Ruohonen K. Preoperative leg length inequality and hip osteoarthrosis: a radiographic study of 100 arthroplasty patients. Skeletal Radiol. 2005;34:136–9.

Greulich WW, Pyle SI. Radiographic evidence of skeletal development of the hand and wrist. 2nd ed. Stanford: Stanford University Press; 1959.

Tanner JM, Whitehouse RH. Clinical longitudinal standards for height, weight, height velocity, weight velocity and stages of puberty. Arch Dis Child. 1976;51(3):170–9.

Westh RM, Menelaus MB. A simple calculation for the timing of epiphyseal arrest: a further report. J Bone Joint Surg Br. 1981; 63-B(1):117–9.

Chapter 14
Skeletal Dysplasia

Sulaiman Alazzawi and Kyle James

Introduction

Skeletal dysplasias are a heterogeneous group of genetic disorders that affect growth, development and maintenance of bone and cartilage. The incidence is estimated to be around 2–5/10,000 live births.

There are more than 450 different types. Approximately 40% of them can be diagnosed at birth while the rest usually manifest later during childhood. There are at least 70 different types that are so severe that survival is limited to the perinatal period. Currently, 226 implicated genes have been identified in 316 different phenotypes. Inheritance can be autosomal dominant, autosomal recessive, X-linked recessive or X-linked dominant and may vary in the degree of severity.

S. Alazzawi, MBChB, MSc, MRCS
T&O SpR Royal London Rotation, London, UK

K. James, FRCS (Tr&Orth) (✉)
Paediatric and Young Adult Orthopaedic Unit,
The Royal London and Barts and The London Children's
Hospitals, Barts Health, London, UK
e-mail: Kyle.James@bartshealth.nhs.uk

N.A. Aresti et al. (eds.), *Paediatric Orthopaedics
in Clinical Practice*, In Clinical Practice,
DOI 10.1007/978-1-4471-6769-3_14,
© Springer-Verlag London 2016

Terminology

Given the breadth of skeletal dysplasias, the terminology is varied. They can be described based on the type of the tissue involved:

- *Osteodysplasia*: Involves bone and can be subdivided into two main types:
    - Osteopenia.
    - Oteosclerosis.

- *Chondrodysplasis*: Involves the cartilage and hence affects the linear growth of the bone, leading to short stature.
- *Osteochondrodysplasias*: Involves both bone and the cartilage.

Alternatively, dysplasias can be described based on the anatomical region of the abnormality, which is commonly used in radiological descriptions (See Table 14.1).

Descriptions can be based on the specific site of limb shortening (see Fig. 14.1):

- Proximal segment: Rhizomelic.
- Middle segment: Mesomelic.
- Distal segment: Acromelic.

Other terms used to describe deformities include:

- Diastrophic = twisted.
- Camptomelia = bent.
- Metatrophic = changing.

TABLE 14.1 Dysplasias, based on the anatomical region of the abnormality

Site	Effect
Epiphyseal	Joint pathologies Short stature
Metaphyseal, diaphyseal	Short, deformed long bones
Spondylodysplasis	Cervical instability Kyphoscoliosis

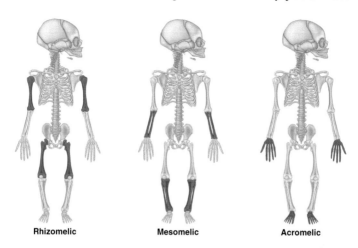

Rhizomelic   Mesomelic   Acromelic

FIGURE 14.1 Anatomic description of skeletal dysplasias

- Thanatophoric = fatal in the neonatal period.
- Platyspondyly = flat vertebrae.
- Achondroplasia = short-limbed.

It is important to remember that the term *dwarfism* is no longer in use, and instead the deformity can be described as a short stature.

Classification

Classifying skeletal dysplasias is similarly difficult owing to the variety in types. Possible classifcations systems include:

- **Clinical**
  - Proportionate: Limb length is approximately the same length as the trunk. This is commonly associated with medical or endocrine conditions such as Turner's syndrome. Two main groups of disorders exist:
    - Cleidocranial dysplasia – recognizable clinical features such as frontal bossing and short middle phalanges, along with absent or partially missing clavicles.

- Mucopolysaccharidoses – Recognised through positive complex sugars in the urine.

- Disproportionate: In general these disorders lead to either a short trunk with normal size limbs (e.g. achondroplasia) or short limbs with a normal size trunk (e.g. Morquio's).

  - Disproportionate short trunk skeletal dysplasias:

    - Kneist's dysplasia: associated with a cleft palate deformity and deafness.
    - Spondyloepiphseal dysplasias: accompanied by spinal deformities.

  - Disproportionate short limb skeletal dysplasias:

    - Achondroplasia: associated with particular facial features, e.g. a large head, frontal bossing, a small midface and flattened nasal bridge.
    - Multiple Epiphyseal Dysplasia: without facial involvement.
    - Osteogenesis imperfecta (OI): altered bone density.
    - Multiple hereditary exostoses: associated with multiple osteochondromas.

- **Radiological**

  - Bone region affected (see Table 14.1).
  - Bone density:

    - Osteopenia.
    - Osteoporosis.

  - Individual structural irregularities:

    - Skull – Wormiam bone in OI.
    - Hypoplastic clavicles (cleidocranial dystosis).

- **Molecular/genetic**

  The majority of skeletal dysplasias can be accounted for by abnormalities in 11 different gene mutation families or broadly characterized in four groups:

- Defects in the structural protein of cartilage: collagen/ cartilage oligomeric matrix protein (COMP).
- Errors in local regulators of cartilage growth: Fibroblast growth receptor, parathyroid hormone related peptide receptor, cell surface heparin sulphate receptor (EXT).
- Errors in cartilage metabolism: Diastrophic Dysplasia Sulphate Transporter.
- Systemic defects influencing cartilage development: lysosomal enzymes.

- **Mendelian inheritance**

  - The majority are autosomal dominant, e.g. Achondroplasia (Fig. 14.2).
  - Autosomal recessive, including some forms of osteo-genesis imperfecta or multiple epiphyseal dysplasia.
  - X-linked, e.g. Hunter's type II MPS.

Diagnosis of Skeletal Dysplasias

Skeletal dysplasias may be diagnosed during the prenatal period, at birth or during childhood. Prenatal diagnosis is predominantly based on the use of ultrasound examination. Despite being a common and routine perinatal assessment, the ultrasound diag-nosis of skeletal dysplasia can be challenging due to the variable presentations of the pathology. Sonographers must have a high index of suspicion when a family history is present. Subtle fea-tures that may suggest the presence of a dysplasia include:

- Unequal bone lengths.
- Absence, hypoplasia or malformation of bones.
- Abnormal chest circumference and cardiothoracic ratio.
- The presence of polydactyly, syndactyly, clinodactyly or any other extremity deformity (see Chap. 4 Hands).
- Abnormal foot length.
- Abnormal head circumference and biparietal diameter.
- The presence of abnormal spinal curvatures (see Chap. 5 Scoliosis).
- Unusual pelvic geometry.

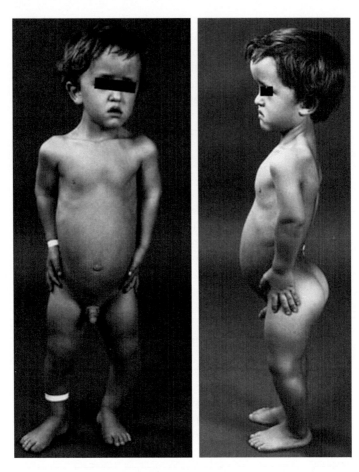

FIGURE 14.2 Achondroplasia. Note the characteristic features described above (Reproduced from Benson et al. *Children's Orthopaedics and Fractures*, 2009, Springer)

Several factors from the parental history and features at birth may aid the diagnosis, or raise suspicion, of a skeletal dysplasia. Such features include:

- Positive family history.
- Maternal age.
- Previous stillbirth.

- Low or high birth weight.
- Length of child.
- Arm span.
- Head circumference.
- Associated congenital malformations, e.g. laryngomalacia, tracheomalacia or bronchomalacia.
- Maternal use of certain medications during pregnancy, e.g. warfarin, which may cause stippled epiphyses.

Skeletal dysplasia may present late, during childhood, with features such as short stature or inappropriate upper/lower segment ratio. Similarly associated abnormalities may prompt a diagnosis, such as hearing and/or visual impairment or connective tissue abnormalities. A radiological assessment at late presentation should include full a skeletal survey and a measurement of bone density. Laboratory tests should include:

- Calcium.
- Phosphate.
- Albumin.
- Alkaline phosphatase.
- Parathyroid hormone.
- Vitamin D.

Other useful investigations include cytogenetic tests, to assess chromosomal deletions or rearrangements, molecular genetic testing and biochemical testing.

Common Orthopaedic Problems Associated with Skeletal Dysplasia

- Spinal disorders: the common spinal disorders that are associated with skeletal dyplasias are:
  - Thoracolumbar kyphosis (70%).
  - Scoliosis (25%).
  - Atlantoaxial instability/cervical kyphosis (15%).
  - Spinal Stenosis.

- Neurological complications associated with such spinal deformities may produce the following clinical features:

    - Gait deterioration.
    - Deterioration of neurological function, i.e. muscle fatigue and hyper-reflexia.

- Limb disorders, including:

    - Joint deformity.
    - Limb malalignment.
    - Arthritis.
    - Soft tissue laxity.
    - Contractures.
    - Limb length discrepancy or overall shortening.

> Atlanto-axial subluxation can lead to sudden death and therefore performing a cervical spine X-ray is essential during assessment of a patient who presents with a skeletal dysplasia.

Management

Assessing the patient is best achieved through a multidisciplinary approach. A detailed family history should be sought, spanning at least three generations, and including any fetal deaths. Examination should include the use of growth charts, measurement of upper to lower segment ratios and a detailed systematic examination to exclude any associated disorders. Routine investigations should include skeletal surveys, biochemical tests, genetic tests and possible histological examination of tissue.

Management Principles

Treatment of SD patients is complicated and generally varies depending on the aetiology, and also on patient factors. Broadly speaking, the orthopaedic goals of treatment are to achieve:

- Relatively normal mechanical alignment of the limbs and spine.
- Prevent neurological compromise.
- Match joint surfaces.
- Correct leg length discrepancy.
- Manage acute fractures.
- Treat variable soft tissue contractures or laxity.

Non-operative treatment options, including physical therapy and orthoses, have been used to varying degrees of success. Orthotic options include casting, bracing and ankle-foot orthoses. They are particularly useful in treating soft tissue and joint laxity in younger children, but often exaggerate the underlying limb or spinal deformity.

The surgical management of limb malalignment is broadly divided into two main strategies. The first is guided growth with the use of staples, or plate and screw fixation, i.e. a (hemi)epiphysiodesis. The expected rate of growth of normal bone is usually 1° per month in the coronal plane and 2° per month in sagittal plane. In dysplastic bone, the rate of correction will often be slower and sometimes the rate of growth is delayed to such an extent that guided growth is not feasible.

The second strategy is the use of corrective wedge osteotomies to treat limb deformity, lengthening or shortening. Managing limb shortening by attempting limb lengthening however, is controversial for skeletal dysplasia patients. In the presence of joint laxity, lengthening of a limb may lead to joint subluxation. Acute fixation or frame techniques can be used to facilitate osteotomies.

The second strategy is a corrective osteotomy to treat limb deformity, which can be stabilised with either internal or external fixation. Managing limb shortening through limb lengthening is controversial for short stature individuals. In the presence of joint laxity, lengthening of the limb may lead to joint subluxation or dislocation.

Certain considerations are required in managing specific disorders of skeletal dysplasia. For example, long bone fractures associated with osteogenesis imperfecta are best treated with intra-medullary devices.

The surgical management of spinal problems includes decompression in cases of spinal stenosis (more commonly at the lumbar region) and posterior instrumented fusion for cervical spine kyphosis and atlantoaxial instability (eg. in Morquio's syndrome).

Common Types of Skeletal Dysplasia

Achondroplasia (Fig. 14.2)

- 20% autosomal dominant inheritance.
- 80% new mutation.
- 1 in 100,000 births.
- Mutation in the FGFR3 (fibroblast growth factor receptor 3), leading to increased inhibition of chondrocyte growth in the proliferative zone of the physis.
- Risk factors include maternal age above 36.
- The clinical picture includes: short stature with limb shortening, frontal bossing, a 'saddle' nose, bilateral genu varum and posterior radial bowing which can lead to posterior radial head dislocation.
- Spinal disorders are common, and include progressive kyphosis, spinal stenosis due to congenital short pedicales (which may require decompression) and narrowing of the foramen magnum (which may lead to sudden death).
- Limb deformities may require corrective osteotomies.

Hypochondroplasia

- This is a less severe form of achondroplasia, which is also autosomal dominant and is also due to a (different) genetic mutation in FGFR3.

Thanatophoric Dysplasia

- Most common lethal dysplasia.
- 1 in 4,000–15,000 births.

- Patients develop severe rhizomelic micromelia.
- A bell shaped chest, depressed nasal bridge and pulmonary hypoplasia are hallmark features.
- There are two types: Type I, where patients have curved femurs, and type II, where there are normal shaped femurs.

Pseudoachondroplasia

- There are four subtypes which are either autosomal dominant or recessive.
- It is caused be an abnormality on chromosome 19.
- There is typically an associated mutation in the gene coding for the collagen oligomeric matrix protein (COMP).
- Clinical manifestations include proportionate dwarfism, short limbs and ligament laxity.
- Pseudoachondroplasia can be differentiated from achondroplasia clinically as pseudoachondroplasics have:

  - A normal face/skull.
  - Normal trunk (other than increased lumbar lordosis).
  - No interpedicular narrowing.

- The child's growth is initially normal and therefore recognition of the disorder tends to be at the around 2–3 year mark.
- Clinical problems include: cervical spine instability, joint laxity and limb malalignment. The latter may ultimately lead to joint arthroplasty.
- Specific features on plain radiographs include small and fragmented epiphyses and cupped, flared, irregular metaphyses.
- Limb lengthening exacerbates joint arthritis.

Osteogenesis Imperfecta

- Osteogenesis imperfecta (OI), the most common skeletal dysplasia, is a group of disorders characterized by defects in type 1 collagen, which is present in multiple tissue types, explaining the varied clinical manifestations.

- Typical clinical features includes:
  - Multiple fractures.
  - Limb deformities.
  - Blue sclera.
  - Scoliosis.
  - Ligamentous laxity.
  - Triangular facies.
  - Macrocephaly.
  - Hearing loss.
  - Defective dentition.
  - Barrel chest.
  - Growth retardation.

- Although the incidence of OI is described as 1 per 20,000 live births, the milder form is under diagnosed and so the incidence may well be higher.
- Diagnosis depends on individual history, family history, examination, blood tests for endocrine and nutritional causes of low bone density, radiological skeletal survey, DEXA scan and rarely genetic testing.
- Although OI is most likely a continuum of disease, the modified Sillence classification (summarised in Table 14.2) is used to categorize OI. Originally it was a phenotypic classification containing four types; however as molecular and genetic understanding has increased it has been expanded to now include 15 types. 90% fall into the Sillence Type I and IV categories. Most OI subtypes are inherited in an autosomal dominant fashion.
- Medical management includes calcium and Vitamin D supplements and the use of bisphosphonates.
- Osteoblastic activity is preserved, therefore fracture healing is not impaired. Most fractures can therefore be treated conventionally.
- Upper limb fractures can be treated non-operatively with lightweight casts. Attention should be made to prevent deformity, which increases the re-fracture rate, and an X-ray should confirm union before cast removal.
- Corrective osteotomies may be required to correct deformities.

TABLE 14.2 Modified Sillence Classification of Osteogenesis Imperfecta (Type 1-V) – listed in order of increasing frequency of deformity and fractures

Type (no of Subtypes)	Inheritance	Eye	Comment
Type I (2)	Autosomal dominant	Blue sclera	Most common Fractures occurs as the child starts to walk, osteoporosis, acetabular protrusio
Type IV (2)	Autosomal dominant	White sclera	Can be confused with NAI Similar to type I but with white sclerae
Type V (1)	Autosomal dominant	White Sclera	Associated with calcification of interosseous membrane, hyperplastic callus Dislocation of radial head
Type III (12)	Autosomal recessive	Pale Blue sclera	Wheelchair bound Progressive bowing fractures Kyphoscoliosis As the lumbar spine shortens, ribcage overlaps the narrow pelvis,
Type II (6)	Autosomal dominant	Blue sclera	Lethal – death within few hours after birth Prenatal ultrasound diagnosis

- Extendible intramedullary rods, such as the Fassier-Duval rod, can be used to treat fractures to minimize re-operation as the patient grows.
- Surgical management of the spine includes decompression for basilar invagination and posterior instrumented fusion for severe thoracic kyphosis due to multiple fracture or scoliosis.

Multiple Epiphyseal Dysplasia (MED)

- MED is a form of dwarfism characterized by delayed ossification of multiple epiphyses (Figs. 14.3 and 14.4).

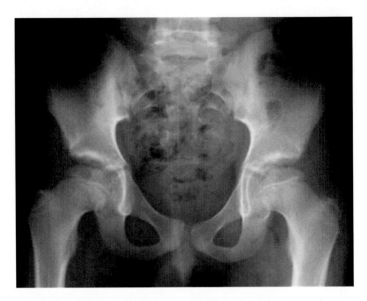

FIGURE 14.3 Multiple epiphyseal dysplasia (MED) of the hips

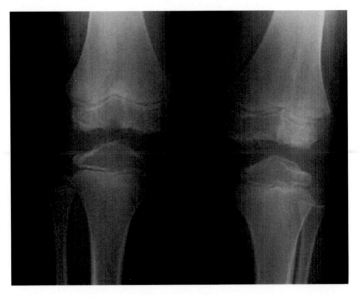

FIGURE 14.4 Multiple epiphyseal dysplasia (MED) of the knees

- The incidence is approximately 1 in 10,000. Like other skeletal dysplasias, MED is a spectrum of disease, which can be autosomal dominant or recessive. Six genes have been identified to be involved, leading to a series of mutations. Most autosomal forms are attributable to a mutation in the gene coding for collagen oligomeric matrix protien (COMP).
- Patients typically present in late childhood with painful and stiff joints (particularly hips and knees), limb malalignment, gait abnormality, early fatigue after exercise, elbow contractures and restricted shoulder movement.
- Differential diagnoses include Perthes' disease, hypothyroidism and storage disorders. An important differentiation is that Perthes' disease tends to be asymmetric whilst MED affects the epiphyses at both hips as well as of other joints.
- Radiographic features include short stunted metacarpals, hyperextensible fingers, double patella & Glacier signs.

Hereditary Multiple Exostosis

- HME is a condition characterized, as its name suggests, by multiple exostoses.
- The incidence is around 1 in 100,000.
- Although it is autosomal dominant, 30% of cases arise as new mutations.
- The genes most commonly effected are EXT1 on chromosome 8, EXT2 on chromosome 11 and EXT3 on chromosome 19.
- The exostoses arise from metaphyseal bone, commonly at the insertion points of tendons, and point away from the epiphyses.
- The common sites of involvement are the distal radius, proximal humerus, proximal femur and around the knee.
- Clinical problems include local bony prominence, compression of adjacent tissue, asymmetrical growth, angular deformity and limb length inequality.

- Malignant changes occur in 0.5–5% (chondrosarcoma), therefore regular long term monitoring is required in high-risk patients.
- Surgery is required to relieve local symptoms such as pain or nerve compression, to re-align joints or to correct leg length discrepancy.

Mucopolysaccharidosis (MPS)

- MPS is a group of glycogen storage disorders characterized by a deficiency of hydrolase enzyme degrading glycosaminoglycans. This leads to an accumulation of mucopolysaccharides and ensuing tissue and organ dysfunction. Some of the more common ones are presented in Table 14.3.
- The most striking orthopaedic clinical features include:

  - Proportionate short stature.
  - Increased rate of carpal tunnel syndrome.
  - Atlantoaxial instability.
  - Delayed hip dysplasia.
  - Bullet-shaped phalanges.
  - Genu valgum.
  - Abnormal epiphyses.

- Patients typically have the following non-orthopaedic features:

  - Ophthalmic disease (e.g. corneal clouding, glaucoma).
  - CNS disease (e.g. hydrocephaly).
  - Cardiorespiratory disease (e.g. valvular dysfunction, pulmonary obstruction, sleep apnoea).
  - Deafness.
  - Cognitive impairment.

- Diagnosis is typically made via urine testing although pre-natal screening is possible through chorionic villus sampling and amniocentesis.
- New treatments such as enzyme replacement therapy and bone marrow transplantation are improving survival and decreasing the need for orthopaedic intervention.

TABLE 14.3 Examples of types of mucopolysaccharidosis

	Syndrome	Inheritance	IQ	Common features
Type I	Hurler	Autosomal recessive	Lower	Characteristic facial appearance Hazy cornea Joint stiffness Kyphosis Death due to respiratory or cardiac complications.
Type II	Hunter	X-linked	Lower	Clear corneas Macrocephaly Coarse facial features Joint contractures
Type III	San Filippo	Autosomal recessive	Lower	Wheelchair-bound at an early age
Type IV	Morquio-Brailsford syndrome	Autosomal recessive	Normal	Common Normal face Short neck Barrel chest Pectus carinatum Short stature Ligamentous laxity – C1 to C2 instability
Type VI	Maroteaux-lamy	Autosomal recessive	Normal	Mild pattern of MP I

Key References

Brown RR, Monsell F. Understanding the skeletal dysplasias. Curr Orthop. 2003;17:44–55.

Kinning E, McDevitt H, Duncan R, Faisal Ahmed S. A multidisciplinary approach to understanding skeletal dysplasias. Expert Rev Endocrinol Metab. 2011;6(5):731–43.

Antsaklis A, Anastasakis E. Skeletal dysplasia. DSJUOG. 2011;5(3):205–12.

Caroline Lois Cheesman Rouin Amirfeyz Martin Francis Gargan. How to approach a patient with skeletal dysplasia. Orthop Trauma. 2014;28(2):97–105.

Dighe M, Fligner C, Cheng E, Warren B, Dubinsky T. Fetal skeletal dysplasia: an approach to diagnosis with illustrative cases. Radiographics. 2008;28(4):1061–77.

Savarirayan R, Rimoin DL. The skeletal dysplasias. Best Pract Res Clin Endocrinol Metab. 2002;16(3):547–60.

Chapter 15
Musculoskeletal Infections

Zacharia Silk and Krishna Vemulapalli

Introduction

Acute septic arthritis is the inflammation of a synovial joint caused by pyogenic organisms, which can result in articular damage, joint deformity and long-term disability if left untreated.

Osteomyelitis is the infection of bone, which can be acute (symptom duration <2 weeks), subacute (typically resulting in a Brodie's abscess) or chronic (symptom duration >6 weeks, with radiological evidence of sequestrum and involucrum).

Epidemiology

Musculoskeletal infection in children is now much less common, with an annual incidence in developed countries ranging from 1.94 to 13/100,000 child population. The incidence of

Z. Silk, MBBS, BSc (Hons), MRCS
T&O SpR Percivall Pott Rotation,London, UK

K. Vemulapalli, MBBS, FRCS, FRCS (Tr&Orth) (✉)
Department of Trauma and Orthopaedics, Barking, Havering and Redbridge Hospitals, London, UK
e-mail: Krishna.Vemulapalli@bhrhospitals.nhs.uk

N.A. Aresti et al. (eds.), *Paediatric Orthopaedics in Clinical Practice*, In Clinical Practice, DOI 10.1007/978-1-4471-6769-3_15, © Springer-Verlag London 2016

septic arthritis is twice as common as osteomyelitis in early childhood, but similar in later childhood. Whilst this decline in incidence is welcome, clinicians are becoming less exposed and, consequently, less experienced in managing this condition.

Risk factors associated with osteomyelitis include a history of blunt trauma in 29.4% patients and recent systemic infection in 37.4%.

Early diagnosis with prompt and effective treatment is more likely to lead to an excellent outcome, and therefore infection must remain at the forefront of one's differential diagnosis when assessing a limping child.

Aetiology

There are three modes of bacterial spread implicated in the development of musculoskeletal infection:

1. **Haematogenous spread**
   In children, this is by far the most common route. It may be caused by distant infection affecting the ears, mouth, respiratory tract, gastrointestinal system, genitourinary system or skin (e.g. infected umbilical cord in neonates, chickenpox in infants).
2. **Local spread**
   Septic arthritis can occur if an adjacent subcutaneous or subperiosteal abscess communicates with the joint. This is more likely at sites where the joint capsule extends to the metaphysis (e.g. hip, ankle, shoulder and elbow joints).
3. **Direct inoculation**
   This can occur due to a penetrating wound (e.g. open fracture) or following a surgical procedure. This is the least likely route of infection in this age group.

Pathology

Transient episodes of bacteraemia can occur at any time (e.g. during the course of a distant infection or following dental work); however a normal host response usually results in spontaneous resolution before the onset of clinical infection.

A balance exists between the virulence of the organism (i.e. the comparative pathogenicity of different organisms), the hosts' response to pathogens and the effect of other contributing factors (e.g. haematoma and/or tissue necrosis following trauma). An organism of low virulence will only cause an infection if a large number of bacteria are present or the host response is impaired, whereas a highly virulent organism requires a much smaller number of bacteria to infect a normal host. Because of this relationship, haematogenous osteomyelitis can take an acute, subacute and chronic path.

We cover the pathophysiology of acute haematogenous osteomyelitis and septic arthritis below. A thorough understanding of the basic pathophysiology helps to explain the radiographic findings of osteomyelitis.

Pathophysiology of Acute Haematogenous Osteomyelitis

1. **Bacterial seeding**
   The sharp hairpin bend in the metaphyseal capillaries lying adjacent to the physis reduces blood flow sufficiently to allow bacterial seeding to take place. This makes the metaphysis the most likely area of a long bone to become infected.
2. **Local inflammation**
   The host response to the presence of bacteria leads to a local increase in vascular permeability, resulting in oedema, increased vascularity and the recruitment of polymophonuclear leucocytes.
3. **Subperiosteal abscess formation**
   Acute inflammation and suppuration within the tight confines of the medullary cavity increases intraosseous pressure, causing pain and an obstruction to arterial and venous blood flow. Pus is exuded through the Volkmann canals to the surface of the bone, where the relatively inelastic periosteal layer becomes elevated.
4. **Avascular necrosis of underlying bone**
   As intraosseous and sub-periosteal pressure further increases, vascular stasis and thrombosis occurs such that the endosteal and periosteal blood supply to the affected

area becomes disrupted and the underlying bone becomes necrotic and begins to resorb. The dead bone becomes fragmented resulting in the formation of sequestra, which provokes a foreign body reaction and makes the eradication of bacteria impossible until it is either extruded from the body or surgically excised. This represents the start of the chronic phase of osteomyelitis.

5. **Subperiosteal new bone formation**
In chronic osteomyelitis, the sequestrum is enveloped by a layer of new bone (involucrum) originating from the deep layer of the periosteum to create a permanent reservoir of infective tissue. This new bone first appears on the radiograph at around 7–10 days. Spontaneous discharge of pus may occur through perforations in the involucrum called *cloacae,* which may form a sinus with the skin if left untreated.

6. **Resolution**
Healing can occur with adequate surgical excision of the necrotic bone and soft tissue and with appropriate antimicrobial therapy.

Special Considerations

1. **The difference between infants and children**
In the young infant, the presence of transphyseal blood vessels can also allow the haematogenous spread of pathogens from the metaphysis into the epiphysis and even the joint, leading to growth plate injury and septic arthritis. After the first year of life, the transphyseal vessels become obliterated and the physis matures, creating a barrier to bacterial spread (see Fig. 15.1).

2. **Chronic & Subacute Osteomyelitis**
Organisms of low virulence may proliferate in patients with an impaired host resistance to cause a subacute or chronic osteomyelitis. In subacute osteomyelitis, a walled off, pus-filled, cavity (i.e. bone abscess or Brodie's abscess)

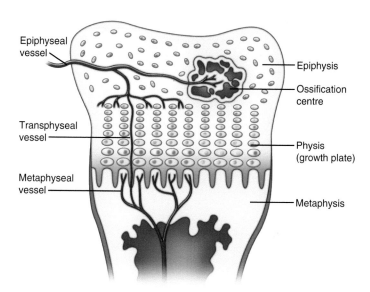

FIGURE 15.1 Open ended hair-pin arrangement of metaphyseal blood vessels adjacent to the physis with transphyseal vessels crossing across into the epiphysis. This arrangement predisposes infants to septic arthritis and growth plate injury. The transphyseal vessels disappear after the first year of life and the physis becomes a barrier to the haematogenous spread of infection from the metaphysis to the epiphysis. (Modified from Benson et al *Children's Orthopaedics and Fractures*, Springer, 2009)

may form. This is usually found in sites of rapid skeletal growth, such as the proximal tibia, distal femur, humeral metaphysis or distal radius. Symptomatically, patients tend to have only mild and intermittent pain in the absence of a systemic inflammatory response.

Chronic osteomyelitis results from an untreated or inadequately treated acute infection, or it may silently bypass the "acute" phase and first come to light after the development of sequestrum, involucrum and a sinus tract.

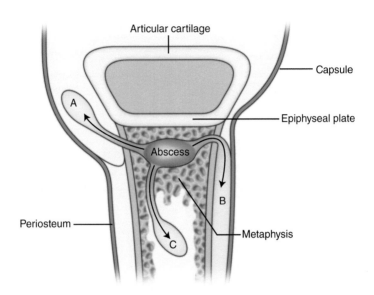

FIGURE 15.2 Showing the spread of pus from a metaphyseal focus of osteomyelitis – (A) directly into the joint, (B) into a subperiosteal abscess, (C) into the medullary canal. (Modified from Benson et al *Children's Orthopaedics and Fractures*, Springer, 2009)

Pathophysiology of Septic Arthritis

1. **Bacterial Seeding**

   This can occur in a number of ways:

   1. Haematogenous spread to synovial capillaries, which form micro-abscesses that rupture into the joint.
   2. Transphyseal vessels present in young infants can permit the spread of bacteria from a metaphyseal osteomyelitic focus into the epiphysis, which can perforate the articular cartilage to enter the joint. The osteomyelitic lesion often becomes apparent several days after the initial presentation of an acute episode of septic arthritis (Fig. 15.2).
   3. Direct inoculation into the joint via a periarticular abscess or trauma.

2. **Local Inflammation**
   An acute synovitic reaction leads to the development of a seropurulent exudate, resulting in a painful joint effusion, which can cause joint subluxation or even dislocation in severe cases. Pus may even burst out of a joint to cause an abscess.
3. **Articular Erosion**
   The presence of bacterial and proteolytic enzymes released by leucocytes leads to a progressive and irreversible erosion of the articular cartilage, and the largely cartilaginous epiphysis.
4. **Epiphyseal Avascular Necrosis**
   Increasing intra-articular pressure further reduces perfusion of the remaining epiphysis, causing avascular necrosis if left untreated.
5. **Healing phase**
   Depending on the timing and success of medical intervention, complete resolution of the infection with a return to normal function can occur. However, delay in treatment may lead to partial loss of articular cartilage with fibrosis of the joint, bony ankylosis and eventual bone destruction, leaving the child with a lasting deformity.

Pathogens Causing Infection

A host of organisms can cause either osteomyelitis or a septic arthritis. Normally between 50% and 75% of organisms are identified. They include:

- Staphylococci – These gram + ve cocci are responsible for the majority of infections. *Staphylococcus aureus* is a constituent of normal skin flora. Many strains are possible and resistance to antibiotics common.
- MRSA – Methicillin Resistant Staphylococcus Aureus is becoming more common and isolated more frequently. It is more common amongst those with risk factors and institutionalised patients.
- Streptococci – Another of the Gram + ve family, the beta haemolytic strain accounts for most cases. It tends to effect neonates or older children.

- *Haemophilus influenzae* – Particularly in populations which do not have an immunization program against it.
- Others – *Escherichia coli, Kingella kingae* and mycobacteria.

Symptoms and Signs

As haematogenous spread is usually the commonest cause of septic arthritis in this group of patients, special attention should be made to investigate for and treat any distant sites of primary infection. The source of infection could arise from a multitude of sites, including the CNS, chest, abdomen, spine, upper respiratory tract, ears, urinary tract and skin, including the umbilical cord or intravenous cannula sites, hence the extra vigilance required when assessing such patients (Table 15.1).

The clinical features of paediatric musculoskeletal infection differ according to age and site.

1. **Neonates** (up to 4 weeks old):
   Newborns tend to have an atypical presentation with few clinical signs. Constitutional symptoms include general irritability and a refusal to feed. This can be associated with or without signs of a systemic inflammatory response syndrome (SIRS). Careful inspection, palpation and movement

TABLE 15.1 Risk factors for the development of musculoskeletal infection

Malnutrition
Sickle cell disease
Immunosuppressive drugs
Diabetes
Immunocompromised states (e.g. HIV infection, Chemotherapy, Steroid use)
Neonates
Postoperative

of the affected limb and/or joint should take account any local inflammatory features, such as subtle signs of effusion (abnormal skin creases; bulge over joint), pain, warmth and resistance to movement.

2. **Infants** (1–12 months) and **children**
   The more typical features of septic arthritis include inability of the patient to bear weight on the affected joint or actively move it (pseudoparalysis) due to the presence of a tense joint effusion and pain. Passive movement of the joint helps to differentiate septic arthritis from the pain caused by osteomyelitis, which does not usually result in painful passive joint movements. There may be overt signs of inflammation, including warmth to touch, swelling and a hyperaemic appearance of the overlying skin. As with neonates, associated signs of a SIRS or sepsis may be present, requiring careful monitoring of the pulse, temperature and hydration status.

Investigations

Targeted investigations can be considered using the following principles:

1. **Look for evidence of a systemic inflammatory response**
   White Cell Count, Erythrocyte Sedimentation Rate (ESR), C-reactive protein (CRP)
2. **Search for a potential source of infection**
   Urine dipstick & mid-stream urine, chest X-ray
3. **Confirm the site of infection**

   1. **Radiographs**
      In osteomyelitis, radiological signs may not be visible until 10–14 days after the onset of clinical infection. Early signs include the presence of lytic lesions, periosteal new bone formation and soft tissue swelling. In septic arthritis, a joint effusion and soft tissue swelling may be visible.
   2. **Ultrasonography**
      This is the main investigation used in the diagnosis of either septic arthritis or a sub-periosteal abscess

associated with osteomyelitis. In cases of septic arthritis, synovial swelling and joint distension can be observed.

3. **Computer Tomography (CT)**

   This can clarify the degree of bone destruction and soft tissue involvement, but is of limited value in the diagnosis and management of acute osteomyelitis/septic arthritis.

4. **Nuclear medicine**

   This is useful in cases of diagnostic uncertainty; when suspecting multifocal disease; or when investigating for infection in unusual sites (e.g. the spine).

5. **Magnetic Resonance Imaging (MRI)**

   MRI has significant advantages over radioisotope scanning due to the absence of ionizing radiation and greater diagnostic specificity when investigating unusual sites, such as the pelvis and spine. The most significant disadvantage, however, is a high likelihood of movement artefact unless the child is adequately sedated or anaesthetised. In the majority of cases of osteomyelitis, MRI is not necessarily required and certainly should not delay treatment if the diagnosis can be proved using simpler means.

4. **Identify a causative organism**

   1. **Blood Culture**

      The false negative rate is high, but in the presence of sepsis, a positive result can be used to guide treatment, especially if the urgency of the clinical situation demands antimicrobial administration before the acquisition of formal microbiological samples. Higher yields of viable organisms may be obtained during episodes of high fever and rigors.

   2. **Joint Aspirate**

      In cases of suspected septic arthritis, a joint aspirate should be performed prior to the administration of antimicrobials to maximise the chance of obtaining a positive culture. Document the fluid's colour and clarity in the notes before sending to the laboratory for urgent Gram stain, culture and sensitivity. It should be noted, however, that approximately 33% of culture positive aspirates have an initially negative gram stain, therefore in view of this high false negative rate, the result of a Gram stain alone should not be relied upon to exclude joint infection. If the culture result is negative, but clinical suspicion remains high, liaise with your microbiologist to request a polymerase chain reaction (PCR) analysis of the sample to help isolate the pathogen.

3. **Pus Sample**

   In cases of osteomyelitis, an ultrasound-guided aspirate of a subperiosteal abscess can be sent for microscopy, culture and sensitivity. If tuberculosis is suspected, ensure the sample is tested for acid-fast bacilli.

4. **Synovial/Bone Biopsy**

   Tissue removed at the time of surgery should also be sent for culture to further assist in the isolation of the offending pathogen.

Monitoring Infections

After initiation of appropriate treatment, observe the patient for clinical signs of recovery, including the resolution of pain, return of movement and the ability to bear weight in a previously pseudo-paralysed limb.

In the clinic, assess the trend of the CRP over time. This is a more sensitive and timely reflection of the acute phase response than the ESR as its rise and fall in response to disease and treatment is much quicker. This will help guide overall length of antimicrobial therapy.

Differential Diagnosis

A number of other conditions may present with bone and joint pain, including malignant, haematological and inflammatory causes.

Examples include:

1. **Transient synovitis** – a recent viral upper respiratory tract infection may precede transient synovitis. Whilst the joint may be painful and the child reluctant to move it, there are

TABLE 15.2 Kocher's clinical predictors for differentiating between septic arthritis/transient synovitis

No of predictors	Transient synovitis	Septic arthritis	Predicted probability of septic arthritis (%)
0	19(22.1%)	0(0%)	<0.2
1	47(54.7%)	1(1.2%)	3.0
2	16(18.6%)	12(14.6%)	40.0
3	4(4.7%)	44(53.7%)	93.1
4	0(0%)	25(30.5%)	99.6

Four predictors: History of fever >38.5 degrees; Non-weight bearing; ESR >40 mm/hr; WBC >12 × 10^9/L

usually no signs of infection, normal inflammatory markers and the child tends to appear well (Table 15.2).

2. **Perthes' disease.**
3. **Slipped capital femoral epiphysis.**
4. **Juvenile idiopathic arthritis** – ask about a personal or family history of autoimmune disease. Pain and swelling is likely to be gradual and the patient is less likely to be systemically unwell.
5. **Psoas abscess.**
6. **Haemophilia** – intra-articular bleeding can result in a tense and painful haemarthrosis, which can significantly limit the child's ability to move the affected limb. Usually the child is systemically well and a joint aspiration along with an analysis of the clotting function would reveal the diagnosis.
7. **Sickle-cell disease** – a sickle cell crisis may lead to avascular necrosis, and can mimic the presentation of septic arthritis. In addition, sickle cell disease can also predispose patients to bone and joint infection. Although *Staphylococcus aureus* is the most common pathogen in the paediatric and sickle population, *Salmonella typhi* is also frequently seen in this cohort (Fig. 15.4).

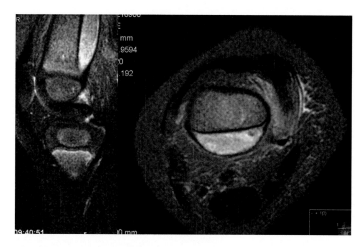

FIGURE 15.3 MRI scan showing a subperisoteal femoral collection

Treatment

The principles of treating any musculoskeletal infection are as follows:

1. Provide analgesia and general supportive treatment.
2. Splint the affected limb/joint.
3. Obtain a microbiological sample.
4. Initiate appropriate antibiotic therapy.
5. Remove pus and necrotic tissue, if required.

Osteomyelitis

Surgical drainage may not be required if the osteomyelitis is detected and treated before the development of a subperiosteal abscess. If pus is evident, however, surgical debridement is indicated and allows a formal microbiological sample (fluid and tissue) to be obtained prior to the initiation of antibiotics. Necrotic tissue should be removed followed by copious

FIGURE 15.4 Plain radiograph of osteo-myelitis in a sickle patient

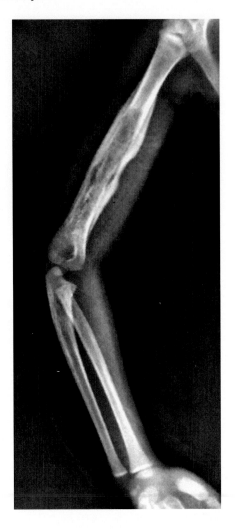

lavage with isotonic saline solution, although the structural integrity of the bone should be maintained.

In refractory cases of chronic osteomyelitis, a more radical excision of the diseased segment of bone is required, followed by reconstruction using a bone transport technique.

Septic Arthritis

Pus in the joint must be evacuated urgently to prevent articular damage. This is more commonly done using an open approach; however, arthroscopic techniques may also be used (e.g. knee/shoulder). Repeated needle irrigation and aspiration may be performed for more superficial joints, although this is not a practical consideration in the vast majority of children who would object to this whilst awake.

In both situations, it is important to preserve function by initiating movement as soon as clinical improvement is seen. Septic joints treated surgically and with antibiotics immediately or within 3 days tend to completely recover.

Follow-Up

Regular outpatient observation of the patient's clinical and laboratory markers of infection is required until such time the patient remains infection-free after a reasonable period of time following the termination of antibiotic therapy. Patients with established chronic osteomyelitis should be informed of the possibility of late recurrence and warned about the need for repeat investigation, should even the most subtle symptom or sign return.

In all cases of septic arthritis and neonatal osteomyelitis, longer-term follow up is required to ensure delayed skeletal complications do not occur.

Complications

Septic Arthritis

1. Dislocation caused by a tense effusion.
2. Destruction of articular cartilage resulting in joint fibrosis, ankylosis and pain.
3. Avascular necrosis of the epiphysis following a significant delay in decompressing a tense joint effusion. This may lead to the formation of a pseudoarthrosis (Tom Smith's dislocation).

Osteomyelitis

1. Adjacent joint infection, either through direct or transphyseal spread.
2. Physeal damage resulting in growth disturbance and/or angular deformity, especially if affecting one of a pair of bones (e.g. forearm/leg).
3. The development of chronic osteomyelitis if treatment is delayed and/or inadequate.

Overwhelming sepsis resulting in multiorgan dysfunction is uncommon, but can be a very serious complication.

Synopsis

Osteomyelitis and septic arthritis are common disorders amongst children. The morbidity is high and the mortality low. Various investigations aid the diagnosis, but frequently it is based on clinical grounds alone. Surgical debridement of an abscess or washout of a septic joint, followed by antibiotics, forms the mainstay of treatment. Kocher's criteria provide a useful tool in differentiating between septic arthritis and transient synovitis.

Key References

Kocher MS, et al. Differentiating Between Septic Arthritis and Transient Synovitis of the Hip in Children: An Evidence-Based Clinical Prediction Algorithm. J Bone Joint Surg Am. 1999; 81(12):1662–70.

McCarthy JJ, et al. Musculoskeletal infections in children. Basic treatment principles and recent advancements. J Bone Joint Surg Am. 2004;86:850–63.

Yeo A, Ramachandran M. Acute Haematogenous Osteomyelitis In Children. BMJ. 2014;348:g66

Dartnell J, Ramachandran M, Katchburian M. Haematogenous acute and subacute paediatric osteomyelitis: a systematic review of the literature. J Bone Joint Surg Br. 2012;94(5):584–95

Chapter 16
Paediatric Musculoskeletal Tumours

Daniel Williams and Krishna Vemulapalli

Definitions

Neoplasia from the Greek 'neo', meaning new and 'plasma', meaning creation. This refers to the pathological process of abnormal, excessive and inappropriate proliferation of cells or tissue.

Benign tumours A group of well-differentiated abnormal cells that lack the ability to invade neighbouring tissue or to metastasize. A benign tumour will remain localised to a single mass and cause symptoms by direct pressure upon adjacent structures.

Malignant tumours A group of poorly differentiated abnormal cells that may invade surrounding tissue and metastasize to distant sites.

D. Williams, MBChB, BSc (Hons), MRCS
T&O SpR Percivall Pott Rotation, London, UK

K. Vemulapalli, MBBS, FRCS, FRCS (Tr&Orth) (✉)
Department of Trauma and Orthopaedics,
Barking, Havering and Redbridge Hospitals, London, UK
e-mail: Krishna.Vemulapalli@bhrhospitals.nhs.uk

N.A. Aresti et al. (eds.), *Paediatric Orthopaedics
in Clinical Practice*, In Clinical Practice,
DOI 10.1007/978-1-4471-6769-3_16,
© Springer-Verlag London 2016

Epidemiology

The majority of benign bone tumours are asymptomatic, often detected as an incidental finding. As such the true incidence is difficult to determine. Malignant bone tumors comprise 3–5% of cancers diagnosed in children 0–14 years and 7–8% in adolescence 15–19. They are very rarely diagnosed in children younger than 5. Although there are more than 20 sub-types of malignant primary bone tumors, greater than 80% are osteosarcoma (52%) or Ewing's sarcoma (34%) [1].

Aetiology

The aetiology of most benign and malignant bone and soft tissue tumours is not known. 20% of children have a family history of the condition, however there are a large number of hereditary and non-hereditary conditions associated with an increased risk. These are mainly caused by genetic alterations of cell cycle constituent genes, such as retinoblastoma syndrome (RB1), genes involved in growth–regulating transcriptional cascades such as enchondromatosis (PTHR1) and multiple hereditary exostoses (EXT1, EXT2).

Pathogenesis

Soft tissue tumours that present to the orthopaedic surgeon can originate the following tissue types:

- Fibrous.
- Lipomatous.
- Neural.
- Muscular.
- Vascular.
- Synovial.

TABLE 16.1 Types of bone tumour

Tissue type	Benign	Malignant
Bone	Osteoid osteoma	Osteosarcoma
	Osteoblastoma	Ewing sarcoma
	Osteochondroma	
Cartilage	Enchondroma	Chondrosarcoma
	Chondromyxoid fibroma	
Fibrous tissue	Fibrous cortical defect	Fibrosarcoma
	Fibrous dysplasia	
	Fibrocartilaginous dysplasia of the tibia	
Miscellaneous	Simple bone cysts	Metastatic disease
	Anuerysmal bone cyst	
	Giant cell tumour	
	Langerhan cell histiocytosis	
	Massive osteolysis	
	Haemangioma of bone	

Bone tumours can be primary bone producing lesions, chondrogenic lesions or fibrous lesions. These are summerised in Table 16.1. There are several tumors of unknown origin such as Ewings and Giant Cell Tumours, as well as tumour-like conditions such as aneurysmal bone cysts, simple bone cysts, Langerhans cell histiocytosis and fibrous dysplasia. Tumours of haemopoetic origin and secondary bony metastases also occur in children.

Symptoms/Signs

Bone tumours commonly present with persistent pain, classically worse at night. Diagnosing 'growing pains' is a common mistake and this should be a diagnosis of exclusion. This is in contrast to soft tissue sarcomas, which commonly manifest as painless masses. Often patients only seek advice when the mass becomes painful, fails to resolve or enlarges.

A history of trauma or persistent pain following a traumatic incident is a common mechanism of presentation. Trauma may raise awareness of lesion, lead to a pathological fracture or a radiograph which itself may result in an incidental finding. There is no evidence that trauma precipitates bone or soft tissue tumours. Tumours may also cause neurological symptoms secondary to compression, erosion or tumours of nerve origin. They may also present with symptoms of metastasis to distant site such as the lung.

Investigations

Diagnosis of the musculoskeletal tumours starts with a good clinical history including family history and clinical examination. Investigations for suspected neoplasia may include any of the following:

Plain Radiographs

Radiographs provide valuable diagnostic information and some tumours have very characteristic appearances. Lesions are described by their location within the bone (diaphyseal, metaphyseal, epiphyseal) and their relationship with the cortex. Lesions may be lytic, sclerotic or demonstrate a mixed pattern. Slow growing tumours generally have a narrow zone of transition with a well-demarcated appearance in comparison to fast growing tumours, which more commonly have a permeative, wide zone of transition ± a periosteal reaction or elevation (endosteal scalloping or Codman's triangle which can be seen in

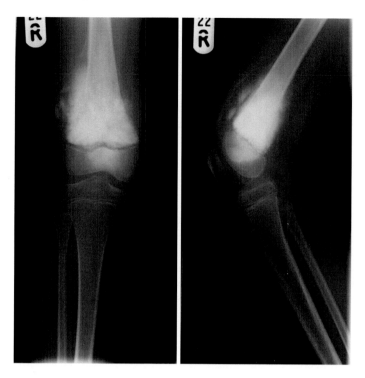

FIGURE 16.1 Plain radiographs demonstrating an extensive densely osteoblastic distal femoral metaphyseal osteosarcoma, which has spread into the central aspect of the epiphysis but does not appear to involve the joint. There is also a circumferential extraosseous extension. A Codman's triangle is also visible

Fig. 16.1). Aggressive tumours may have cortical erosion (scalloping) where as slower growing tumours may result in bony expansion.

Cross Sectional Imaging & Scintography

Magnetic resonance imaging (MRI) and computerised tomography (CT) allow detailed information on local and distant staging. MRI can identify when tumours cross compartments, clarify the extent of oedematous change, the relationship to neurovascular structure and joints as well as identifying skip lesions. Positron emission tomography (PET CT) can help assess tumor activity and metabolism, differentiate between benign and malignant tumours, plan operative procedures, monitor response to chemotherapy and help to predict a patient's prognosis. Bone scintography and radionuclide scanning can be useful in detecting small lesions, skip lesions or metastases.

Biopsy

Histological specimens can be gained through incisional, percutaneous or excisional biopsy. Primary malignant bone tumours are complex and rare and, as such, should be managed at regional specialist centres to minimise the chance of incomplete excisional biopsy and ensure the incision/tract is well planned and marked so that it can be excised when the tumour is removed. A biopsy should only be performed after appropriate cross sectional imaging has been undertaken as the biopsy can lead to haemorrhage, fracture or infection, which could significantly alter the diagnostic accuracy.

Percutaneous biopsy can be performed via a core biopsy or fine needle aspiration cytology (FNAC). They are commonly performed under image guidance to avoid a necrotic core and a non-diagnostic specimen. Histological analysis, immunohistochemistry and cytogenetics can achieve excellent diagnostic accuracy. Samples in the form of fresh specimens should be sent urgently to specialist centres as certain decalcification protocols can reduce the diagnostic accuracy.

Blood Tests

Blood tests may be important in the diagnosis, establishing a baseline prior to potent cytotoxic therapy as well as guiding prognosis such as alkaline phosphatase in osteosarcoma.

TABLE 16.2 Enneking staging of bone tumours

Grade:

G1 – Low grade, moderate cytological atypical and a low risk of metastasis,

G2 – High grade, high mitotic rate, necrosis and microvascular erosion. There is a higher risk of metastasis.

Tumour size:

T1 – Intracompartmental

T2 – Extracompartmental

Metastasis:

M0 – No metastasis

M1 – Metastasis present

Stage 1A = G1, T1, M0

Stage 1B = G1, T2, M0

Stage 2A = G2, T1, M0

Stage 2B = G2, T2, M0

Stage 3 = M1

Classification Systems

Despite the rarity of bone tumors there is a very wide spectrum of entities. Classification is based on the recognition of the dominant tissue, the architecture, and type of matrix produced by the tumor.

Soft tissue tumours are staged using the Enneking Staging system; G = histological grade (1–3), T = Size, N = Lymph node involvement and M = Metastasis (Table 16.2).

Differential Diagnosis

A number of conditions may mimic a tumour clinically or radiographically. The common differentials include:

- Infection.
- Soft tissue haematoma.
- Myositis ossificans.
- Stress fracture.
- Tendon avulsion injuries.
- Medullary infarcts.

Treatment Principles

1. Treatment should be in a tertiary centre specialising in the management of bone and soft tissue tumours.
2. Benign and asymptomatic lesions make up the majority of bone tumours in children. Such cases often do not require any treatment if there is diagnostic certainty.
3. Benign bone tumours may be painful or enlarging. Once the diagnosis has been confirmed, they can be appropriately treated, usually by resection or curettage.
4. Treatment of malignant tumours is dependent of the site and grade. Lesions can be excised through an intra-lesional approach (debulking, low risk of recurrence), marginal excision, wide excision, radical excision (tumour is excised as a block without exposing the lesion), or amputation.
5. The treatment of a tumour should not be at the expense of the prognosis. However, with advances in technology, improved methods of imaging and advances in adjuvant therapy, limb salvage procedures are increasingly being used. In growing children, extendible implants can reduce the need for repeat operations. Grafting and distraction osteosynthesis are also suitable in some instances.
6. (Neo)adjuvant therapy: In sensitive tumours neoadjuvant or adjuvant multi-agent chemotherapy can reduce the size of primary lesions, prevent metastatic seeding and improve survival. Radiotherapy is occasionally used in highly sensitive tumours although in a restricted manner. Complications such as pathological fracture, post irradiation spindle cell sarcoma and soft tissue trauma limit its use. The main use is following marginal excision, in

combination with chemotherapy in high-grade tumours or inoperable tumours due to their size, inaccessible location, advanced local spread or proximity to major blood vessels.

Malignant Tumours

Osteosarcoma (Fig. 16.1)

Osteosarcomas make up 3% of all childhood cancers. The majority occur in the second decade of life. The most common sites for osteosarcoma in children are the distal femur, proximal tibia and humerus. There are many sub-types with the most prevalent being the "common type" – high-grade intramedullary osteosarcoma. 90% of intramedullary high-grade lesions have a cortical breach at presentation (stage IIb) and 10–20% have distant metastasis. Neoadjuvant chemotherapy has been shown to improve survival and following wide margin surgical resection. The overall 5-year survival rate is 71% in children.

Ewing's Sarcoma (Fig. 16.2)

80% of Ewing's sarcomas are diagnosed in childhood with a mean age of 13. The femur, pelvis and proximal humerus are the most common sites. Ewing's usually presents with pain and constitutional symptoms such as fever and weight loss. Radiographs often show a large destructive lesion with a significant soft tissue component. The classical radiographic appearance is that of the periosteum being lifted off in layers producing an onion-skin like appearance.

Multi-modality individualised approach to treatment with multi-agent chemotherapy, radiotherapy and surgical resection all play an important role. With current treatment, the overall 5-year survival rate for localized disease at presentation is around 70%. When the cancer has already spread at presentation the 5-year survival rate is around 15–30%.

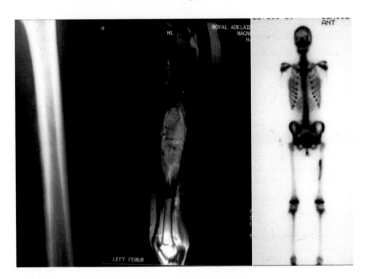

FIGURE 16.2 Ewing's sarcoma plain radiograph, MRI and bone scan

Benign Tumours

Osteoid Osteoma (Fig. 16.3)

These are tumours consisting of osteoblasts, vascular tissue and thin-faced osteoid seams. They are diaphyseal cortically based and appear as an area of lucency surround by a sclerotic margin. They are often difficult to see on plain radiographs. Osteoid osteomas are more common in males (2:1) and appear from as early as the age of 5. Symptoms include pain that is worse at night and with alcohol consumption, but relieved by NSAIDs. When peri-articular, they may mimic arthritis. They may be treated with NSAIDs alone, radiofrequency ablation or surgery.

Osteoblastoma

These are histologically similar to osteoid osteomas although they have more giant cells. They are mainly differentiated by their size (>1.5 cm as opposed to smaller than), their

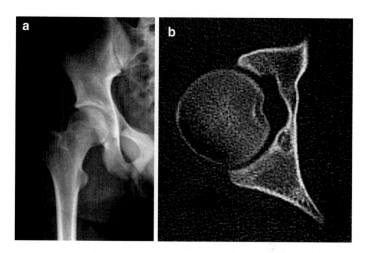

FIGURE 16.3 Plain radiograph (**a**) and axial CT (**b**) of an osteoid osteoma of an acetabulum. Notice the difficulty in seeing it on the plain radiograph whereas on the axial CT, a lucent lesion with sclerotic and reactive margins can be seen

propensity for posterior spinal elements and metaphyseal regoins of long bones and their more aggressive manner. They should be treated surgically.

Osteochondroma (Figs. 16.4 and 16.5)

These are very common benign bone tumours that are formed following endochondral ossification of peri-physeal aberrant cartilage. They commonly occur at the origin of tendons. They may cause local irritation, at which point excision may be warranted. Multiple Hereditary Exostosis is an autosomal condition categorized by multiple osteochondromas with a high risk of malignant transformation to chondrosarcoma (5–10%).

Enchondroma

Enchondromas are benign cartilaginous tumours composed of hyaline cartilage, located in the medullary cavity, typically

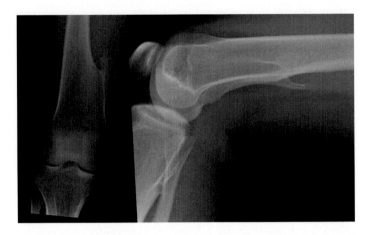

FIGURE 16.4 An AP and lateral radiograph of a distal femur showing two osteochondromas, at the site of the adductor insertions

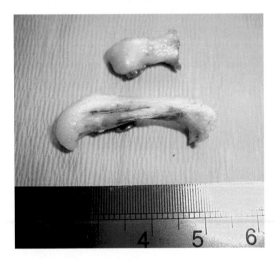

FIGURE 16.5 The excised osteochondroma specimens

of the bones of the hand. Chondroblasts and fragments of epiphyseal cartilage escape from the physis and form the tumours. Multiple tumours are seen in Ollier's disease (Fig. 16.6) and Maffucci's syndrome.

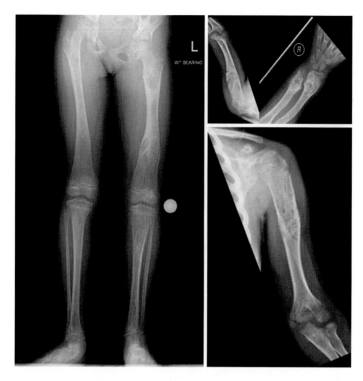

FIGURE 16.6 A selection of radiographs from a patient with Ollier's disease. Notice the multiple enchondromatosis effecting diaphyseal and metaphyseal segments. In some areas the lesions stop proximal to the physis whereas elsewhere the physis is crossed. There is resultant leg length discrepancy and pelvic tilt

Fibrous Cortical Defect/Non-ossifying Fibroma (Fig. 16.7)

These two very common lesions are histologically identical fibrogenic lesions, fibrous cortical defects being smaller than 2 cm and non-ossifying fibromas being larger than 2 cm. They typically appear at the distal femoral junction between the metaphysis and diaphysis and represent well-defined, oval and lucent lesions with a well-demarcated, thin, sclerotic border.

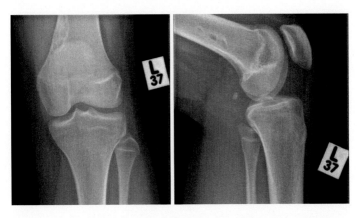

FIGURE 16.7 AP and lateral radiographs of a non-ossifying fibroma: There is a well-defined cortically based lobulated lesion in the medial aspect of the left distal femur with no periosteal reaction or cortical breach

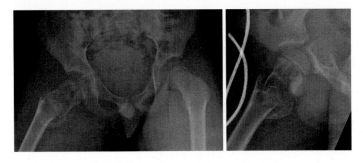

FIGURE 16.8 This is an AP and lateral radiograph of a fracture through a simple bone cyst. Note the large lucent lesion within the metaphysis, which appears slightly expansile and lies adjacent to the epiphysis. The lateral radiograph also has the "fallen-leaf sign"

Simple (Unicameral) Bone Cysts (Fig. 16.8)

These are very common clear serosanguineous fluid filled lesions, surrounded by a fibrous membranous lining. They appear as well defined lesions with a narrow zone of transition. The surrounding bone may have expanded, leading to thin cortices. Importantly, there is no periosteal reaction or soft tissue swelling. Over half occur in the proximal humerus and they commonly present following a fracture through them. Following a fracture, a pathologic sign is a cortical fragment that has fallen within the cyst ('fallen leaf' sign). Active lesions are located adjacent to the physis, and occasionally go through it. Latent lesions have a bridge of bone between the physis and cyst. Lesions may be left alone, aspirated and injected with methylprednisolone or curettaged and grafted (the latter is contraindicated in active lesions as it may affect the physis, leading to growth arrest).

Aneurysmal Bone Cysts (ABC's) (Fig. 16.9)

These tumours may occur at any age although they are most common amongst teenagers. They consist of blood, macrophages, giant cells, and osteoid tissue or bone trabeculae. They typically appear in the metaphysis of long bones, although they may appear anywhere. They are expansile,

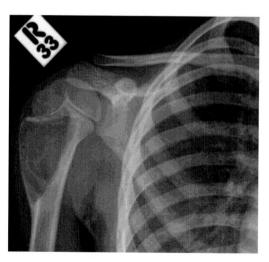

FIGURE 16.9 Aneurysmal bone cyst of the proximal humerus. Notice the explansile, osteolytic lesion with well defined and sharp edges

eccentric, lytic lesions with thin, well demarcated sclerotic borders, giving a 'bubbly appearance'. If they expand quickly, they may lift the adjacent periosteum relative to the normal bone (Codman's triangle). The trabeculae give the appearance of fluid levels on CT/MRI. They either occur primarily or in association with another tumour. Symptomatic ABC's are treated with curettage and bone grafting. If they present following a pathological fracture, they should be treated once the fracture has united.

Synopsis

Paediatric musculoskeletal tumours are diverse, and fortunately malignant tumours are uncommon. The remit of this paper is not to provide an exhaustive text for all tumor types, but a structure by which to assess, evaluate and manage these often complex patients.

Historical Note

James Stephen Ewing (1866–1943) was the first Professor of pathology at Cornell University. Dr. Ewing was co-founder of the American Association for Cancer Research in 1907 and one of the pioneers of using of radiation therapy for cancer. In 1920 he presented perhaps his most famous work on a new kind of malignant osteoma, which later received his name.

Key Reference

Eyre R, Feltbower RG, Mubwandarikwa E, Eden TO, McNally RJ. Epidemiology of bone tumours in children and young adults. Pediatr Blood Cancer. 2009;53(6):941–52.

Index

N.A. Aresti et al. (eds.), *Paediatric Orthopaedics in Clinical Practice*, In Clinical Practice, DOI 10.1007/978-1-4471-6769-3
© Springer-Verlag London 2016